Hemodynamic Monitoring
for Critical Care

Hemodynamic Monitoring
for Critical Care

Debra Bustin, B.N., M.D.
Department of Internal Medicine
University of Calgary
Former Assistant Head Nurse and
Clinical Development Nurse
Intensive Care Unit
Calgary General Hospital
Calgary, Alberta, Canada

 APPLETON-CENTURY-CROFTS/Norwalk, Connecticut

0-8385-3705-7

Copyright © 1986 by Appleton-Century-Crofts
A Publishing Division of Prentice-Hall

88 89 / 10 9 8 7 6 5 4

Prentice-Hall of Australia, Pty. Ltd., Sydney
Prentice-Hall Canada, Inc.
Prentice-Hall Hispanoamericana, S.A., Mexico
Prentice-Hall of India Private Limited, New Delhi
Prentice-Hall International (UK) Limited, London
Prentice-Hall of Japan, Inc., Tokyo
Prentice-Hall of Southeast Asia (Pte.) Ltd., Singapore
Whitehall Books Ltd., Wellington, New Zealand
Editora Prentice-Hall do Brasil Ltda., Rio de Janeiro

Library of Congress Cataloging-in-Publication Data

Bustin, Debra.
  Hemodynamic monitoring for critical care.

  Bibliography: p.
  Includes index.
  1. Pulmonary artery—Catheterization. 2. Patient monitoring. 3. Critical care medicine. 4. Cardiac output—Measurement. 5. Heart—Diseases—Diagnosis. 6. Hemodynamics. I. Title. [DNLM: 1. Critical Care. 2. Heart Catheterization. 3. Hemodynamics. 4. Monitoring, Physiologic—methods. WG 106 B9823h]
  RC683.5.P84B87 1986   616'.028   86-1199
  ISBN 0-8385-3705-7

Design: M. Chandler Martylewski
Cover design: Jean Sabato-Morley

PRINTED IN THE UNITED STATES OF AMERICA

In memory of my father, Wilfrid (Bill) Isaac

Contents

Preface

Hemodynamic monitoring involves the observation of how the cardiovascular system responds to illness, injury, and therapeutic intervention. It includes both invasive and noninvasive methods of assessing cardiovascular performance. In this book we shall be discussing those hemodynamic parameters obtained through the use of flow-directed balloon-tipped pulmonary artery catheters.

This book is intended for use by critical care clinicians who have basic knowledge of hemodynamic measurements made with pulmonary artery catheters, and who have had some clinical experience using these catheters. Its purpose, therefore, is not to concentrate on presenting basic information to beginning practitioners, but rather to build on previous knowledge and experience in critical care and thereby promote personal and professional growth plus optimum patient care.

The book has been developed in three sections:

Section 1. Review of Cardiovascular Structure and Function
Section 2. Determination of Cardiac Output and Derived Hemodynamic Parameters
Section 3. Clinical Applications of Hemodynamic Measurements

Each section is followed by a quiz to test your comprehension of the material covered. Quiz answers are provided at the end of each section. These quizzes can also be used as pretests prior to working through each section. Section 3 contains a series of case studies with questions designed to provide practice in the correlation and assessment of hemodynamic changes associated with various clinical conditions and in evaluation of the effectiveness of therapeutic interventions affecting ventricular function.

This book has benefited greatly from suggestions offered by many reviewers. I wish, in particular, to thank Dr. John V. Tyberg, Departments of Internal Medicine and Medical Physiology at the University of Calgary, for his valuable assistance. I would also like to extend my thanks to Mr. Don Whiting, Mr. Nairne Douglas, and

Mr. Jerry Groves for their assistance in obtaining waveform tracings, and to Ms. Linda Corbeil, who diligently typed the manuscript. Special thanks to my husband, my family, and many dear friends for their support and encouragement throughout this endeavor.

A Note from the Author

Intensive-care units utilize an abundance of sophisticated equipment in providing care for the critically ill patient. Hemodynamic monitoring plays an essential role in patient assessment and in determination of appropriate therapeutic interventions. It is necessary to remember, however, that there is a person beneath this technology and that sophisticated equipment can never replace the "human touch." Close patient observation by the bedside clinician remains the most important assessment tool; invasive hemodynamic monitoring is an adjunct that, when integrated with information from observations, laboratory data, and other sources, helps us provide optimum patient care and management.

Review of Cardiovascular Structure and Function

This section consists of a brief review of cardiovascular structure and function. The information presented forms the basis for understanding hemodynamic changes. This is not intended to be comprehensive; it is merely a review, emphasizing those principles pertinent to understanding hemodynamics.

MYOCARDIAL CELL STRUCTURE AND FUNCTION

Cardiac muscle is composed of myocardial cells, also called myocardial fibers. These myocardial fibers have multiple branches, dividing and recombining to form an interconnecting network. The boundaries between individual fibers, referred to as intercalated discs, have very low impedance to electrical impulses, allowing rapid transmission of these impulses throughout the myocardium (Fig. 1–1).

The network structure of myocardial fibers, along with the presence of the low-resistance intercalated discs, allows the heart to function as a *syncytium*. This means that when an electrical impulse excites one myocardial fiber, the resulting wave of depolarization spreads over the entire network of myocardial fibers. Since the atria are separated from the ventricles by fibrous connective tissue, two separate syncytia exist within the heart—the atrial syncytium and the ventricular syncytium. The atrioventricular (AV) node bridges the atria and the ventricles and allows electrical impulses to be transmitted from atria to ventricles. The significance of the structure of cardiac muscle is that stimulation of any atrial myocardial fiber causes depolarization of the entire atrial myocardium and, if the AV node is functional, the impulse will continue on to

1

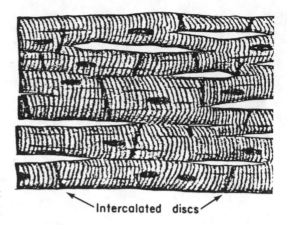

Figure 1–1. The arrangement of myocardial fibers.

Intercalated discs

cause depolarization of the ventricular myocardium as well. Similarly, stimulation of any ventircular fiber will cause depolarization of the entire ventricular myocardium.

Myocardial fibers are made up of *sarcomeres,* which are the basic contractile unit of the heart. Sarcomeres are composed of actin and myosin filaments, contractile proteins in an overlapping parallel arrangement (Fig. 1–2).

Small structures called *crossbridges* protrude from the surface of the myosin filament. These crossbridges can interact with the neighboring actin filaments, causing the actin to slide along the myosin filament. This results in shortening of the sarcomere and contraction of the myocardium. Actin filaments contain troponin and tropomysin proteins, which regulate the interaction between the actin filament and the crossbridges of the myosin filaments (Fig. 1–3).

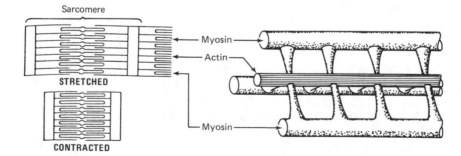

Figure 1–2. Schematic representation of a myocardial sarcomere, showing the parallel arrangement of myosin and actin. *(Adapted from Langfitt D: Critical Care Certification and Review. Bowie, Md: Brady, 1984, p. 107.)*

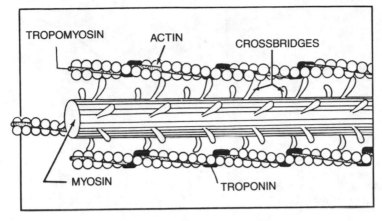

Figure 1–3. Schematic representation of myosin and actin interaction, showing myosin crossbridges, and the troponin and tropomyosin regulatory proteins on the actin filament. *(Adapted from Langfitt D: Critical Care Certification and Review. Bowie, Md: Brady, 1984, p. 106.)*

Calcium ions (Ca^{2+}) must be present before contraction can occur. When the myocardial cell is stimulated, a small influx of Ca^{2+} from the *extracellular* space occurs during the action potential. This slow inward Ca^{2+} channel triggers the release of *intracellular* Ca^{2+}, which is stored in the sarcoplasmic reticulum. With

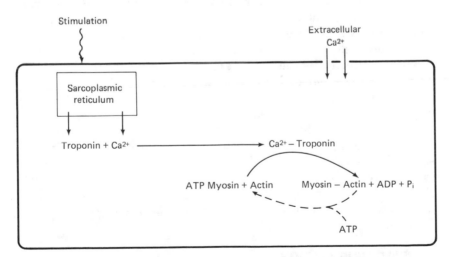

Figure 1–4. Influx of extracellular Ca^{2+} that occurs during the action potential triggers the release of intracellular Ca^{2+} from the sarcoplasmic reticulum. Ca^{2+} attaches to the troponin on the actin filament, enabling the actin and myosin filaments to interact and contraction occurs. ATP is broken down during this reaction. Relaxation occurs when Ca^{2+} is removed from troponin and is pumped back into the sarcoplasmic reticulum.

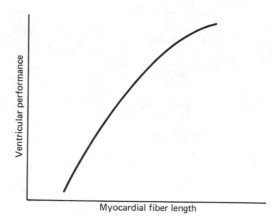

Figure 1–5. Illustration of Starling's law of the heart.

the intracellular concentration of Ca^{2+} increased in these ways, Ca^{2+} attaches to the troponin molecules on the actin filaments, enabling the myosin crossbridges to interact with the actin, and allowing contraction to occur. Calcium ions play an important role in activating the breakdown of adenosine triphosphate (ATP) to provide the energy necessary for myocardial contraction (Fig. 1–4).

The function of the sarcomere is the basis for the Frank–Starling phenomenon, also known as *Starling's law of the heart.*[1] Starling's law involves the ability of the ventricle to vary its force of contraction according to the length of the myocardial fiber just prior to contraction.[17] The essence of Starling's law is that the ventricle can contract with greater force (up to a limit) when the myocardium is stretched before contraction occurs. Myocardial fiber length, i.e., stretch, is affected by the amount of blood within the ventricle just prior to systole (*ventricular end diastolic volume*) (Fig. 1–5).

The relationship between myocardial fiber length and force of contraction can be compared to snapping an elastic band. If the elastic band is stretched slightly and released, it only snaps slightly. The more the elastic band is stretched before release, the stronger it snaps. There is, of course, a limit. If the elastic band is stretched excessively, it will become overstretched and will lose some force. This occurs in the heart as well, where prolonged overstretching of the myocardial fibers results in decreased contractility.

CARDIAC INNERVATION

The heart has an intrinsic electrical system that is able to generate its own electrical impulse to initiate depolarization of the atrial and ventricular myocardium. The autonomic nervous system, however, plays a significant role in regulating the formation and conduction of electrical impulses in the heart. It also influences myocardial contractility.

Sympathetic Innervation

Sympathetic fibers are found throughout the heart; in the sinoatrial (SA) node, atrioventricular (AV) node, and throughout the atria and ventricles. These fibers originate in the upper thoracic spinal cord. Stimulation of the sympathetic fibers causes the release of catecholamines (e.g., norepinephrine), which act on β_1 sympathetic receptors in the myocardial tissue. Stimulation of these β_1 receptors results in an increase in the rate of discharge of the SA node (positive chronotropic effect), an increase in the rate of AV conduction (positive dromotropic effect), and an increase in the force of contraction (positive inotropic effect) of both the atria and the ventricles.

Parasympathetic Innervation

Parasympathetic fibers are found primarily in the SA and AV nodes and the atria, with only a few fibers extending to the ventricles. They originate in the medulla oblongata and extend to the heart via

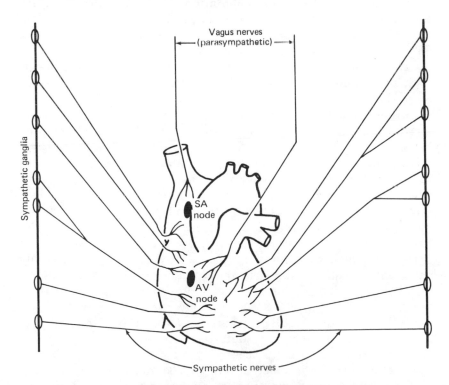

Figure 1–6. Sympathetic and parasympathetic innervation of the heart.

the vagus nerve (cranial nerve X). Vagus nerve stimulation results in the release of acetylcholine, which acts on parasympathetic receptors in the heart. Acetylcholine decreases the rate of discharge of the SA node and inhibits conduction through the AV node. Parasympathetic stimulation has little effect on ventricular contractility and only an indirect effect on ventricular rate (Fig. 1–6).

CORONARY CIRCULATION

The left and right coronary arteries originate just above the aortic valve in the aortic sinuses. They lie on the epicardial surface of the heart and penetrate the myocardium before terminating on the endocardial surface of the heart. The right coronary artery supplies the right atrium, right ventricle, and part of the inferior surface of the left ventricle. It also supplies the SA node in 55% of the population and the AV node in 90% of the population. In approximately 70% of the population the posterior descending coronary artery is the terminal branch of the right coronary artery and supplies the posterior third of the septum and the posterior wall of the left ventricle. The remainder of the population are "left dominant," with the posterior descending coronary artery originating as a branch of the left circumflex artery. The left coronary artery bifurcates to form the left anterior descending (LAD) and the left circumflex (LCA) arteries. The LAD supplies the septal and anterior myocardium of the left ventricle and the LCA supplies the lateral myocardium (Fig. 1–7).

Approximately 75% of the blood flow through the coronary arteries occurs during diastole, when the aortic valve is closed and the aortic sinuses fill with blood. Diastolic pressure, therefore, has a direct effect on coronary blood flow. Collapse of the coronary arteries, with resulting decrease in coronary blood flow, can occur when diastolic pressure falls below 40 mmHg.[12] Coronary blood flow can be further reduced by obstruction of the coronary arteries with atheromatous plaques or by spasm of the coronary arteries. For these reasons, it is important that a diastolic arterial blood pressure of over 40 mmHg is maintained in critically ill patients, especially those with cardiovascular diseases. (A more precise way of determining coronary perfusion pressure is discussed in Section 2.)

Duration of diastole is also an important factor in coronary blood flow. Diastole usually accounts for two thirds of the length of a cardiac cycle, allowing adequate time for ventricular filling and coronary artery perfusion. Excessively rapid heart rates result in a very short duration of diastole and inadequate time for coronary artery filling. Oxygen and nutrient supply to the heart is then re-

ANTERIOR VIEW

POSTERIOR VIEW

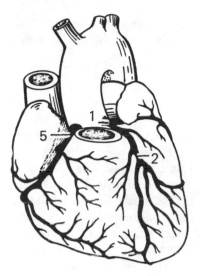
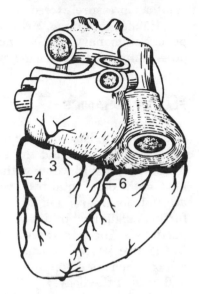

Figure 1–7. The course of the coronary arteries. 1. Left coronary artery. 2. Anterior descending branch. 3. Circumflex branch. 4. Marginal branch. 5. Right coronary artery. 6. Posterior descending artery.

duced at a time when myocardial oxygen demand is increased; this imbalance can lead to ischemia.

PULMONARY CIRCULATION

Pulmonary vessels are significantly different from their systemic counterparts. Pulmonary arteries have thinner walls; specifically, the medial muscle layer is much thinner. Because of this, the resistance in the pulmonary vasculature is approximately one-sixth to one-seventh that of the systemic (peripheral) vascular system.[1] This means that the pulmonary circulation can accommodate a three- to fourfold increase in blood flow before there is any increase in pressure in the system. It follows, then, that an increase in pulmonary artery pressure is more significant than the same change in systemic pressure, as the change in blood flow needed to produce the increased pulmonary pressure is larger than the change required to cause the same increase in systemic pressure.

The pulmonary arteries are low-pressure vessels with the mean pressure normally less than 20 mmHg. In comparison, the systemic arteries are high-pressure vessels, with mean pressures normally 80 to 100 mmHg. Pulmonary edema does not occur until pulmonary capillary pressure exceeds 25 mmHg.

Pulmonary vascular resistance increases in the presence of hypoxia, pulmonary emboli, pulmonary fibrosis, emphysema, and other pulmonary pathologic processes.

FLUID MECHANICS

Body water exists in two main compartments—the intracellular fluid compartment and the extracellular fluid compartment. The intracellular fluid exists within the cells of the body and accounts for two thirds of total body water. The extracellular compartment accounts for the remaining one third of total body water and can be further subdivided into the intravascular and interstitial fluid compartments. The intravascular compartment includes the fluid within the arteries, veins, capillaries, and heart while the interstitial compartment is made up of fluid that surrounds the blood vessels and cells of the body.

Fluid passes easily between the capillaries and the interstitial space, but the volume of each compartment remains constant under normal circumstances. The constant volume is a reflection of the balance that exists between the forces of hydrostatic and oncotic pressures.

Hydrostatic pressure is the pressure exerted by water within each compartment. Since the water within the blood vessels is circulating under pressure, the intravascular hydrostatic pressure is much higher than that in the low-pressure interstitial space. Capillary hydrostatic pressure is further elevated when venous pressures rise, as occurs when the right ventricle fails. If hydrostatic pressure were the only controlling force on fluid within the blood vessels, water would continue to leak out into the interstitium, leading to edema and intravascular hypovolemia.

Oncotic pressure, also known as colloid osmotic pressure, is the pressure exerted by proteins within the fluid compartments. These particles act as water magnets, tending to keep fluid within the blood vessel and drawing in fluid from the interstitial space. Normally, capillaries are impermeable to these proteins, which are retained within the vasculature, and the concentration of proteins within the blood vessels exceeds the concentration in the interstitial space, with the result that water moves inwards. If oncotic pressure were the only force acting on the blood vessels, fluid would be continuously drawn into the vessels, leading to fluid overload and interstitial dehydration.

With both hydrostatic and oncotic pressures acting within the vascular system, a balance is established and equilibrium exists between water lost by the force of hydrostatic pressure and water gained by the force of oncotic pressure. There is a small excess of fluid lost from the intravascular space but this is normally returned to the vascular system via lymphatic flow.

When we discuss pulmonary and systemic vascular pressures, we are talking mainly about hydrostatic forces. It should be clear that when these pressures are elevated to the point where they significantly exceed oncotic pressure, fluid will leak into the interstitium—and we have the occurrence of pulmonary and peripheral edema.

If oncotic pressure drops below normal levels due to loss of protein related to burns, starvation, and so on, pulmonary and peripheral edema can occur despite normal hydrostatic pressure. If the capillaries become "leaky" (i.e., permeability increases) and allow proteins to pass into the interstitium, the problem is compounded. Not only will intravascular oncotic pressure decrease, but fluid will actually be drawn into the interstitium by the proteins that serve to increase interstitial oncotic pressure.

THE CARDIAC CYCLE

Just prior to systole, the ventricles are filled with blood. As the ventricles begin to contract, pressure within the ventricles rises. This rising pressure causes the mitral and tricuspid valves to close, producing the first heart sounds (S_1) and marking the onset of systole. As the ventricular pressure continues to rise it exceeds the pressure within the pulmonary artery and aorta, causing the pulmonic and aortic valves to open. Blood then flows into the pulmonary artery and aorta and the pressure in these vessels increases to its peak or systolic pressure. As ventricular ejection decreases, pressure decreases until the pulmonic and aortic valves again close, producing the second heart sound (S_2). The closure of these valves signals the onset of diastole, when ventricular relaxation begins and the pressure within the ventricles begins to fall until it is lower than the pressures within the atria. This allows the mitral and tricuspid valves to open, and blood again empties from the atria into the ventricles.

Blood flow into the ventricles actually occurs in two phases. The initial (early diastolic) phase accounts for approximately 80% of ventricular filling. In this phase, blood flow is passive and is due to the pressure gradient between the atria and the ventricles. A decrease in ventricular compliance during this initial filling phase may be manifested as an additional heart sound, known as S_3. S_3 is

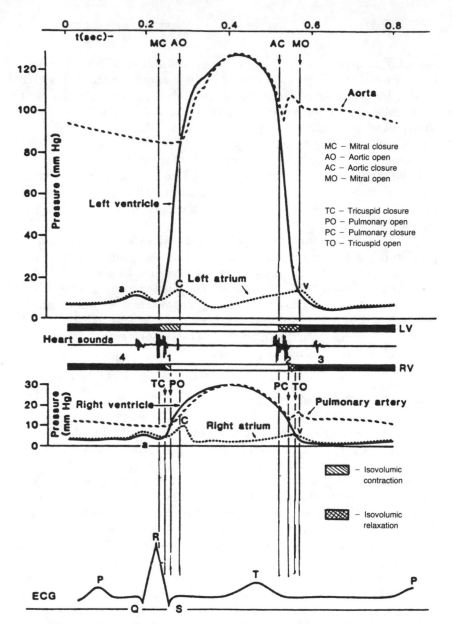

Figure 1–8. Modified Wigger's diagram illustrating the events of the cardiac cycle. Simultaneous right atrial, right ventricular, and pulmonary artery pressure waveforms represent right-sided cardiac events. Left atrial, left ventricular, and aortic pressure waveforms represent left-sided cardiac events. ECG and heart sounds are shown simultaneously to demonstrate their correlation with pressure changes in the various chambers. Note that there is a brief period when the ventricles are contracting against closed semilunar valves (i.e., between MC and AO in the left ventricle and between TC and PO in the right ventricle). This is referred to as *isovolumic contraction*. A brief period of *isovolumic relaxation* occurs after ventricular systole. (*From Milnor WR: In Mountcastle VW (ed): Medical Physiology, 14th edition. St. Louis, Mo: C. V. Mosby Co, 1980, with permission.*)

also referred to as the *ventricular gallop* and may be associated with congestive heart failure where the left ventricle has an already increased end systolic volume and is therefore less compliant when faced with additional blood volume during early diastole.

The second phase of ventricular filling occurs later in diastole and is associated with contraction of the atria, often referred to as *atrial kick*. The atrial kick delivers the remaining 20% of blood to the ventricles. If there is a slight reduction in ventricular compliance, this last bolus of blood may result in a fourth heart sound, known as S_4. S_4 is also referred to as the *atrial gallop* (since it is associated with atrial kick) and may indicate changes in compliance, such as might occur with myocardial infarction.

Both S_3 and S_4 heart sounds are created in the ventricles and are thought to occur due to vibrations resulting when blood flows into the ventricles, whose stretched walls vibrate (resonate) at an audible frequency.

Figure 1–8 shows correlation of the various heart sounds with the events of the cardiac cycle.

INTRACARDIAC PRESSURE CHARACTERISTICS

Normal pressures within each chamber of the heart have definite characteristics that are manifested as specific waveforms when monitored.

Right-sided Cardiac Pressures

Right-sided cardiac pressures are frequently monitored in individuals with cardiac disease. There are no valves between the vena cavae and the atria; therefore, indwelling central venous catheters that are used to obtain central venous pressure (CVP) also reflect right atrial pressure. Swan–Ganz-type pulmonary artery catheters are equipped with a proximal lumen that opens into the right atrium, allowing measurement of right atrial pressure. The distal port of the pulmonary artery catheter allows measurement of pulmonary artery pressure (Fig. 1–9).

Right Atrial Pressure. The atria are the lowest in pressure of all the chambers of the heart. They are also the only chambers to produce waveforms with three positive deflections during the cardiac cycle.

As shown in Figure 1–10, the a wave occurs at the time of the P-R interval and indicates atrial contraction. A decrease in pressure occurs immediately after atrial contraction and is followed by the c wave, which indicates upward movement of the tricuspid valve during ventricular contraction. This is followed by the x descent, which corresponds to atrial relaxation. The v wave corresponds to the T-P interval of the ECG. It represents right atrial filling while the tricuspid valve is closed and is fundamentally related to the accumulation of blood into the closed atrium. The pressure decline following the v wave, known as the y descent, represents the opening of the tricuspid valve and the subsequent blood flow out of the atrium into the ventricle. Sometimes these various atrial waves are difficult to clearly visualize. Mean right atrial pressure ($\overline{\text{RA}}$) measurement is normally used instead of measuring atrial systolic and diastolic pressures, because of the small difference between systolic and diastolic pressure in the atrium.

Normal mean right atrial pressure ($\overline{\text{RA}}$): *0* to *6* mmHg

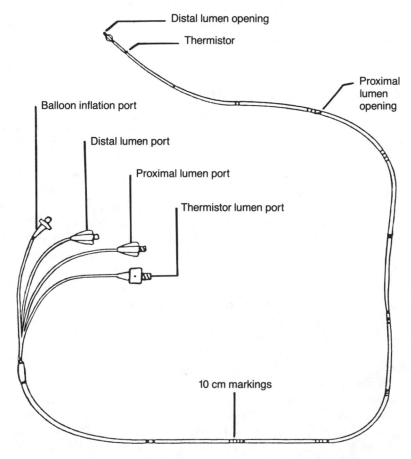

Figure 1–9A. Schematic illustration of thermodilution equipped Swan–Ganz-type pulmonary artery catheter.

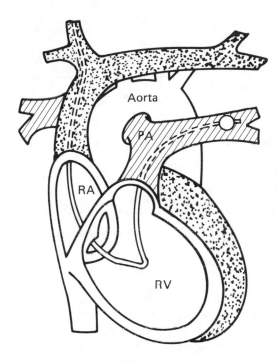

Figure 1-9B. Schematic illustration of pulmonary artery catheter in place within the heart and pulmonary artery.

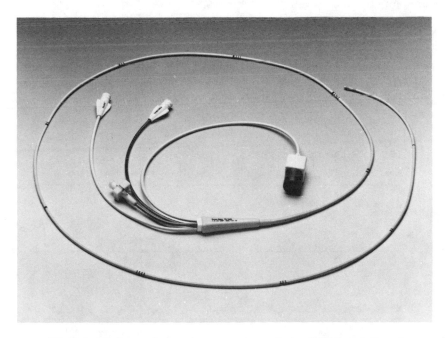

Figure 1-9C. Swan-Ganz pulmonary artery catheter. *(With permission of American Edwards Laboratories.)*

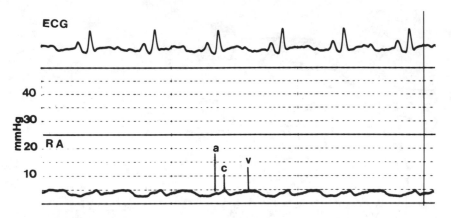

Figure 1-10. RA pressure waveform showing a, c, and v waves. Simultaneous ECG is shown.

Right Ventricular Pressure. The ventricles generate pressures much greater than those found in the atria. For this reason the magnitude of the waveforms is greater for ventricular pressures than for atrial pressures. Ventricular diastolic pressure is almost equal to the mean atrial pressure since the atrium and ventricle are actually a common chamber when the tricuspid valve is open during diastole.

The rapid rise in pressure shown in Figure 1-11 corresponds to early ventricular systole, when the ventricle is contracting against the closed pulmonic valve. When ventricular pressure finally exceeds pulmonary artery pressure, the pulmonic valve opens and ejection of blood into the pulmonary artery causes a gradual de-

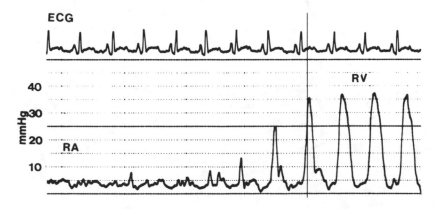

Figure 1-11. Tracing showing RA pressure waveform and change to RV pressure as catheter is advanced. Simultaneous ECG is shown.

crease in pressure in the right ventricle. When pressure in the pulmonary artery exceeds that in the right ventricle, closure of the pulmonic valve occurs, followed by a rapid decrease in pressure as the ventricle relaxes during diastole. Ejection of blood into the pulmonary artery corresponds to the Q-T interval on the ECG. Right ventricular end-diastolic pressure (RVEDP) is measured just before systole begins.

Normal RV systolic pressure: *20* to *30* mmHg
Normal RVEDP: *0* to *6* mmHg (should be approximately equal to $\overline{\text{RA}}$)

Pulmonary Artery Pressure. The pressure in the pulmonary artery during diastole differs from that in the right ventricle (RV). The closure of the pulmonic valve allows the pressure in the RV to fall while pulmonary artery (PA) pressure remains relatively high (Fig. 1–12).

The steep rise in pressure seen in Figure 1–12 represents the ejection of blood into the pulmonary artery from the right ventricle. The pressure then gradually decreases until the pulmonic valve closes. This closure creates the *dicrotic notch* on the PA waveform and marks the onset of diastole. Pressure within the pulmonary artery continues to decline until the next cardiac cycle. Note that while pulmonary artery systolic pressure is normally equal to right ventricular systolic pressure, the closure of the pulmonic valve contributes to the fact that pulmonary artery diastolic pressure is not as low as the ventricular diastolic pressure. Pulmonary artery diastolic pressure is higher than is right ventricular diastolic pres-

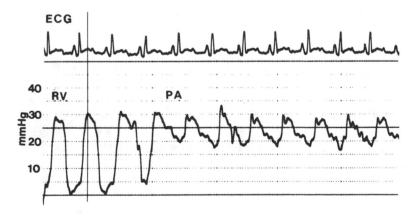

Figure 1–12. Tracing showing RV pressure waveform and change to PA pressure waveforms as catheter is advanced. Simultaneous ECG is shown.

sure, while the PA systolic pressure is the same as RV systolic pressure.

Normal PA systolic: *20* to *30* mmHg (same as RV systolic)
Normal PA diastolic: *6* to *10* mmHg
Normal mean PA ($\overline{\text{PA}}$): < *20* mmHg

Left-sided Cardiac Pressures

Current techniques in hemodynamic monitoring make it possible to obtain important information about left ventricular function without needing to catheterize the left side of the heart. This information is obtained indirectly as the pulmonary capillary wedge pressure (PCWP).

Left-sided cardiac pressures are directly obtainable but these procedures are usually limited to the cardiac catheterization lab. Patients who have undergone open heart surgery may have catheters inserted directly into the left atrium for left atrial pressure monitoring. Measurement of cardiac output using the thermodilution technique (see Section 2) cannot be accomplished using a left atrial catheter, so pulmonary artery catheters are used after cardiac surgery in patients requiring ongoing cardiac output assessment.

Swan–Ganz-type pulmonary artery catheters are the most frequently used method of determining left-sided pressures, and the PCWP approximates the characteristics of left atrial pressure and left ventricular end-diastolic pressure (LVEDP). For these reasons this discussion will be limited to the indirect measurement of LVEDP using PCWP monitoring. It is important to remember that while the pressure waveforms from the left side of heart resemble the corresponding waveforms from the right side, the left side is a higher-pressure system. Figure 1–8 gives a comparison of right versus left-sided cardiac pressures.

Pulmonary Capillary Wedge Pressure The left ventricle is the major pumping chamber of the heart. Left ventricular function is an indication of overall cardiac performance. LVEDP is a major determinant of left ventricular function, as it has a direct effect on myocardial fiber length during diastole, i.e., Starling's law (see section on Myocardial Cell Structure and Function). LVEDP reflects the compliance of the left ventricular myocardium during diastole and the left atrial filling pressure required in order to fill the left ventricle with blood prior to systole.

Figure 1–13 is a diagram of the chambers of the heart and pulmonary circulation during ventricular diastole. Note that there

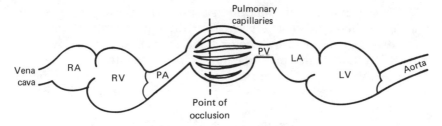

Figure 1–13. Representation of the chambers of the heart and the pulmonary circulation during diastole. The point of occlusion when obtaining wedge pressure is illustrated. Note that the occlusion occurs in one branch of the pulmonary artery, which is in parallel with many other branches, so obstruction of all flow to the lungs does not occur.

is no obstruction between the pulmonary artery and the left ventricle during diastole since the mitral valve is open, so pressures are able to equilibrate at this point in the cardiac cycle. Thus pulmonary artery diastolic pressures can be representative of LVEDP. So why bother using wedge pressures if PA diastolic pressures closely reflect LVEDP? Primarily because PA pressures, both systolic and diastolic, are affected by the compliance of the pulmonary artery, which can be altered by disease states that may not alter LV pressures.

In the patient with normal lungs, the effect of pulmonary artery compliance on PA diastolic pressure is negligible. However, many critically ill patients do have some form of increased pulmonary vascular resistance; many are on positive pressure ventilators, have some form of lung disease, and so on, all of which increase pulmonary resistance. To obtain a more accurate reflection of LVEDP, it is necessary to block out the effects of pressure from the right side of the heart and pulmonary circulation. This is accomplished by inflating the balloon of the pulmonary artery catheter. The catheter then advances until the balloon occludes a small branch of a pulmonary artery, blocking off blood flow from the right side of the heart into that vessel. The pressure obtained distal to the occlusion is the PCWP and is a more direct and reliable reflection of LVEDP.

There are situations, however, in which PCWP is not an accurate reflection of LVEDP.[7] These factors must be kept in mind when assessing a patient's wedge pressure. PCWP is greater than LVEDP in

- Mitral valve disease
- High intraalveolar pressure (e.g., patient on ventilator)
- Pulmonary venous obstruction
- Left atrial prolapsing tumor (myxoma)

These conditions all compromise the open pathway between the wedged catheter and the left ventricle during diastole. Remember: the pressures obtained by wedging the pulmonary artery catheter reflect left ventricular pressure during diastole only, i.e., when the mitral valve is open. The presence of mitral valve disease therefore affects the PCWP accuracy as a reflection of LVEDP; this is discussed in detail in Section 3.

PCWP is also abbreviated as PAW (pulmonary artery wedge), PAWP (pulmonary artery wedge pressure) and PA_o (pulmonary artery occlusion pressure).

The PCWP waveform is a low-amplitude waveform similar to RA and LA tracings. An a wave occurs during left atrial contraction and a v wave occurs, representing filling of the closed atrium during left ventricular contraction. In PCWP or LAP waveforms, c waves are rarely seen (Fig. 1–14). PCWP is measured as a mean pressure value.

Normal mean PCWP: 4 to 12 mmHg

Right–Left Pressure Gradient
The determination of right–left pressure gradient is a simple way to ascertain whether the hemodynamically monitored patient has a pulmonary component to his or her high PA diastolic pressure. This gradient is calculated by subtracting the PCWP from the PA diastolic pressure. The normal gradient is 0 to 6 mmHg.[11] A gradient of greater than 6 mmHg indicates that the patient has a pulmonary problem, i.e., increased pulmonary vascular resistance caused by chronic obstructive pulmonary disease (COPD), adult respiratory distress syndrome (ARDS), hypoxia, pulmonary embolism, and so on. A normal gradient in the presence of elevated PA diastolic pres-

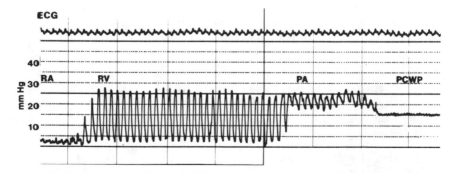

Figure 1–14. Tracing showing pressure waveforms during progression of pulmonary artery catheter from RA through RV and PA to PCWP. Simultaneous ECG is shown.

sure indicates that pump failure or fluid overload is responsible for the high PA pressures.

Some patients will show a mixed picture of pulmonary problems and pump failure or fluid overload. PA values for these patients will show elevated PA diastolic and PCWP plus a right–left gradient of greater than 6 mmHg.

EXAMPLE 1:

A patient is admitted to the Coronary Care Unit (CCU) after an acute anterior myocardial infarction (MI). PA and PCWP values for this patient are:

PA systolic:	38 mmHg
PA diastolic:	25 mmHg
PA:	29 mmHg
PCWP:	21 mmHg

The R-L gradient is $25-21 = 4$ mmHg (normal). PA values and PCWP arc elevated. This indicates that the patient's high PA pressures are due to pump failure or fluid overload, with no pulmonary component.

EXAMPLE 2:

A patient is admitted to the Intensive Care Unit (ICU) with a diagnosis of chronic obstructive pulmonary disease. Her PA and PCWP values are:

PA systolic:	50 mmHg
PA diastolic:	30 mmHg
PA:	37 mmHg
PCWP:	10 mmHg

The R-L gradient is $30 - 10 = 20$ mmHg (abnormally high). PA pressures are elevated but PCWP is within normal limits. This indicates that her high PA values are related to a pulmonary problem.

EXAMPLE 3:

A patient with left ventricular failure develops a pulmonary embolus. PA and PCWP values are

PA systolic:	50 mmHg
PA diastolic:	30 mmHg
PA:	37 mmHg
PCWP:	20 mmHg

The R-L gradient is $30 - 20 = 10$ mmHg (abnormally high). PA pressures are elevated, as in the PCWP. This indicates a problem with both cardiac and pulmonary components.

In general, the presence of an elevated R-L gradient will give an indication of whether there is a pulmonary cause for high PA pressures.

NOTE: PA diastolic pressure cannot be lower than PCWP. This would result in a negative gradient and thus *backwards* blood flow (from LV to PA). Since pressures do vary from beat to beat, a PCWP higher than the PA diastolic may reflect this variation. It may also indicate overwedging of the catheter, where overinflation of the PA catheter balloon results in falsely elevated PCWP readings.

ARTERIAL PRESSURE

Determination of arterial blood pressure is commonly used to assess the cardiovascular status of patients. A brief review of a few important principles of arterial pressure is presented.

Systolic pressure is the highest pressure occurring within an artery during the cardiac cycle. Systolic pressure is affected by factors that regulate diastolic pressure and pulse pressure.

Diastolic pressure represents the lowest pressure occurring in an artery during the cardiac cycle. It is primarily determined by the amount of vasoconstriction present in the arterioles. Increased vasoconstriction will result in an increased diastolic blood pressure while vasodilation of the arterial vasculature results in decreased diastolic pressure.

Pulse pressure is the difference between systolic and diastolic pressure (normally 40–60 mmHg). It is determined mainly by stroke volume and the elasticity of the aorta. A decrease in pulse pressure due to hypovolemia tends to be compensated for by an increased diastolic pressure (increased vasoconstriction). Systolic blood pressure may not fall until blood volume falls significantly below normal.

Mean arterial pressure represents the average pressure within the arterial system during the cardiac cycle. Mean arterial pressure can be estimated by the following formula[18]:

$$\frac{SBP + 2DBP}{3}$$

where SBP is the systolic blood pressure and DBP is the diastolic blood pressure. Diastolic pressure is multiplied by 2 because the diastolic phase of the cardiac cycle lasts twice as long as the systolic phase and we are looking for average pressure over the entire cardiac cycle. Because duration of diastole decreases as heart rate increases, this formula loses accuracy as the heart rate rises over 120 beats/min.

A mean arterial pressure (MAP) of at least 60 mmHg is normally required to maintain tissue perfusion. Mean arterial blood pressure is primarily determined by cardiac output and peripheral (systemic) vascular resistance (SVR). This relationship is illustrated by the following equation:

$$MAP = SVR \times CO$$

(In reality MAP − $\overline{RA}$ pressure = SVR × CO, but since $\overline{RA}$ pressure is usually small compared to MAP, $\overline{RA}$ pressure can be ignored unless it is drastically elevated.)

Thus, changes in cardiac output or systemic vascular resistance will alter blood pressure. For example, an increase in systemic vascular resistance, as might occur with sympathetic nervous system stimulation, would increase mean arterial pressure. An increase in cardiac output would also increase MAP. Decreases in either SVR or cardiac output would decrease mean arterial pressure. The relationship is not quite that simple, however. An increase in SVR will tend to decrease cardiac output since the heart will have to pump against more resistance, resulting in a lesser increase in MAP. The regulatory mechanisms that affect arterial blood pressure will be reviewed in the following section.

REGULATION OF HEMODYNAMIC PERFORMANCE

Cardiac Regulation

There are many regulatory mechanisms that affect cardiac hemodynamics. These mechanisms are aimed at optimizing cardiac output in the presence of stress on the system.

Cardiac output (CO) is the product of stroke volume (SV) and heart rate (HR). This relationship is illustrated in the equation:

$$CO = HR \times SV$$

A change in either HR or SV will alter cardiac output.

Heart Rate. Heart rate changes are the most rapid and effective means of altering cardiac output. Heart rate responds rapidly to signals from

- Sympathetic nervous system. The sympathetic nerves to the SA node release norepinephrine, which increases heart rate.
- Parasympathetic nervous system. Vagal fibers to the SA node release acetylcholine, which decreases heart rate.

- Circulating catecholamines (epinephrine and norepinephrine) released from the adrenal medulla act on SA node to increase heart rate.
- Distention of the right atrium due to overfilling with blood stretches the SA fibers and increases heart rate.

An increase in heart rate can cause a two- to threefold increase in cardiac output. However, excessive increase in heart rate, especially in the critically ill patient, can have undesirable effects. Rapid heart rates increase the oxygen demands of the myocardium (MVO_2) and also decrease the duration of diastole, shortening the time of coronary blood flow and reducing the filling time and hence the amount of blood entering the ventricle prior to contraction.

Just as increased heart rate can increase cardiac output, a decrease in heart rate can cause a decrease in cardiac output. The heart can compensate for this, to a point, by increasing stroke volume via the Starling mechanism (see page 4).

Figure 1–15 illustrates the effect of volume changes on heart rate, stroke volume, and cardiac output.

When intravascular volume is depleted, cardiac output falls. Heart rate increases and the fall in cardiac output is attributed to a

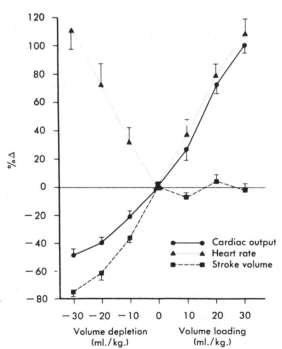

Figure 1–15. Effects of volume depletion and volume loading on cardiac output, heart rate and stroke volume. *(From Vatner SF, Boettcher DH: Circ Res 42:557, 1978, with permission of the American Heart Association, Inc.)*

decrease in stroke volume. When intravascular volume is augmented above normal, the resulting increase in cardiac output is due to an increase in heart rate, as stroke volume remains unchanged.

Stroke Volume

Stroke volume is determined by a combination of three factors:

1. *Ventricular end-diastolic pressure,* also referred to as *preload.* Preload is the effective distending or filling pressure of the ventricle. Although preload is approximated as ventricular end-diastolic pressure clinically, true preload is actually *transmural* pressure. Transmural pressure is the pressure inside the ventricle (end diastolic pressure) minus the pressure outside of the ventricle (pericardial pressure). Conventionally the pericardial pressure has been considered negligible and so has been disregarded when estimating preload. Recent research, however, suggests that this might not be the case, and that pericardial pressure may be more significant than previously thought.[16]

   Preload affects myocardial fiber length and therefore influences force of contraction via Starling's law of the heart. An example of the action of this compensatory mechanism can be seen during a period of decreased heart rate. When heart rate decreases, the duration of diastole is increased. This allows increased time for the ventricle to fill with blood, resulting in increased end-diastolic volume. This increases myocardial fiber length, which enhances force of contraction and results in increased stroke volume.

   In addition to duration of diastole and increase in filling time, there are other factors that influence preload. Diastolic filling pressure, total blood volume, distribution of systemic blood volume, and atrial kick (atrial systole) all affect preload and can therefore influence stroke volume.

2. *Afterload* or resistance to systolic ejection of blood out of the ventricle. This resistance is determined primarily by the tension in the walls of the arterioles. (Afterload can be measured as systemic vascular resistance—see page 54). As resistance to blood flow increases, stroke volume decreases. Figure 1–16 depicts the inverse relationship between stroke volume and afterload at constant preload and contractility. Causes of increased resistance include hypertension, aortic stenosis and autonomic constriction of arterioles. Methods of decreasing afterload can be used to increase stroke volume in patients with left ventricular failure.

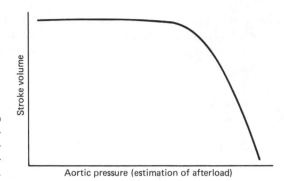

Figure 1–16. The relationship between stroke volume and afterload (as estimated by systolic aortic pressure) at constant preload and contractility.

3. *Contractility,* or the ability of the myocardium to contract effectively. Contractility increases when epinephrine stimulates the β_1 receptors in the heart. If, at fixed ventricular end-diastolic volume, the force of contraction increases, it is said that "contractility" has increased. Contractility is also under direct sympathetic nervous system control. Adrenergic receptors in the myocardium respond to sympathetic stimulation by increasing the force of contraction.

Mild hypoxemia can increase cardiac output indirectly by increasing sympathetic stimulation but severe hypoxemia decreases contractility and decreases cardiac output. Myocardial contractility can be decreased by hypercapnia (Pco_2) and metabolic acidosis. Myocardial injury and infarction effectively decrease ventricular contractility because the resulting scar tissue does not contract, leaving a smaller total amount of myocardial contractile tissue. Furthermore, the normal muscle becomes less efficient because it must stretch the infarcted muscle as well as eject blood.

Disturbances in electrolyte balance also effect contracility. Hyperkalemia ($\uparrow K^+$) and hyponatremia ($\downarrow Na^+$) both exert negative effects on contractility. Hypercalcemia ($\uparrow Ca^{2+}$) increases the force and duration of myocardial contraction.

Pharmacologic agents can both increase (positive inotropic effect) and decrease (negative inotropic effect) contractility. The use of specific inotropic agents is discussed in Section 3.

Other Factors Influencing Cardiac Function

1. *Blood viscosity*
   a. *Anemia.* Decreased blood viscosity produces decreased resistance to blood flow, therefore increasing cardiac output. The heart can maintain adequate oxygen supply to the body tissues in this manner until hematocrit drops well below normal.

b. *Polycythemia.* Increased viscosity results in increased resistance to blood flow, reducing cardiac output. Significant decreases in cardiac output can occur with significantly elevated hematocrits.
2. *Electrolyte imbalance.* As discussed earlier, electrolyte disturbances can alter myocardial contractility. Electrolyte imbalance can also impair cardiac function by causing arrhythmias which slow heart rate, eliminate atrial kick (e.g., complete AV block), or otherwise interfere with effective pumping.

Systemic Vascular Regulation

The systemic (peripheral) vascular system is regulated by local autoregulation and by autonomic nervous system control.

Local autoregulation plays an important role, but it is only partially understood, and may be influenced by local metabolic tissue demands. Oxygen concentration in the peripheral tissues can play a regulatory role. Increased local oxygen concentration produces vasoconstriction whereas decreased local oxygen concentration results in vasodilation. Other factors influencing local blood flow include tissue metabolic needs in relation to nutrient availability. If metabolic demand increases or nutrient supply decreases, vasodilating substances such as lactic acid and bradykinins are released and local blood flow increases.

Nervous system control is accomplished primarily via the vasomotor center in the medulla oblongata, which exerts *sympathetic* effects. This vasomotor center receives signals from many complex mechanisms, including:

1. *Baroreceptors.* These receptors are located in the aortic arch and in the carotid sinuses. They detect changes in arterial blood pressure, to which they respond by altering inhibition of the vasomotor center. This results in changes in vascular tone and arterial blood pressure. An example of this mechanism occurs when the baroreceptors in the carotid sinus sense hypotension. This results in a reflex stimulation of the sympathetic nervous system. Peripheral vasoconstriction results, increasing blood pressure. At the same time, this sympathetic stimulation tends to increase the rate and force of cardiac contraction, which further increases blood pressure.
2. *Chemoreceptors.* These receptors are located in the aortic and carotid bodies and respond to changes in arterial oxygen and carbon dioxide content by influencing the vasomotor center. For example, when the chemoreceptors detect a significant decrease in arterial oxygen tension (Po_2) the vasomotor center may be stimulated to initiate a vasoconstrictive response.

3. *Hypothalamus.* The vasomotor center is signaled by the hypothalamus in response to changes in body temperature, resulting in peripheral vasoconstriction if stimulated in the presence of decreased temperature, or vasodilation if inhibited in the presence of increased temperature.
4. *Venous system.* The venous system also has a regulatory function. Since the walls of the veins are highly distensible, the veins can act as capacitance vessels. For example, if a patient experiences a sudden increase in vascular volume, the tension in the walls of the veins decreases, allowing more blood to be contained in the veins at an only slightly increased pressure. (Of course an increase in hydrostatic pressure would also shift fluid into the interstitial space, causing edema.) Conversely, the tension in the walls of the veins increases if the patient sustains a hemorrhage, thus tending to maintain venous pressure even though there is less blood contained than normal.
5. *Kidneys.* The kidneys also assist in regulation of the cardiovascular system. When blood pressure or blood flow to the

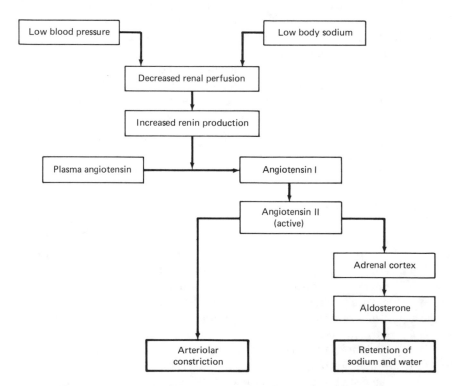

Figure 1–17. Schematic illustration of the renin–angiotensin system.

kidneys decreases, the kidneys respond via activation of the renin–angiotensin–aldosterone mechanism. The release of renin from the kidneys catalyzes the conversion of plasma angiotensinogen to angiotensin I, which is subsequently activated by conversion to angiotensin II. Angiotensin II helps increase blood pressure in two ways. First, angiotensin II is a powerful vasoconstricting agent, which causes vasoconstriction of arterioles throughout the body. This increase in systemic vascular resistance tends to result in an increase in blood pressure. Secondly, angiotensin II stimulates the production of aldosterone by the adrenal cortex. Aldosterone acts on the kidneys to cause retention of salt and water. The resulting increase in intravascular volume also increases blood pressure (Fig. 1–17).

It must be remembered that the aim of these regulatory mechanisms is to maintain homeostasis and, above all, to ensure adequate circulation to the vital organs despite stress on the system.

Summary of Important Concepts in Section 1

1. *Starling's law of the heart* states that the ventricle can contract with greater force (up to a limit) when the myocardium is stretched (myocardial fiber length increased). This can be accomplished by increasing the amount of blood within the ventricle at the end of diastole. However, prolonged overstretching (chronic dilation) of the myocardial fibers results in decreased force of contraction.

2. *Sympathetic innervation* extends to the SA and AV nodes, atria, and ventricles, and stimulation of cardiac β_1 sympathetic receptors results in increased heart rate and increased contractility. *Parasympathetic innervation* is primarily in the SA and AV nodes and atria. The parasympathetic nervous system has little effect on ventricular contractility and only an indirect, albeit very important, effect on ventricular rate.

3. Seventy-five percent of *coronary blood flow* occurs during *diastole*. The faster the heart rate, the shorter the duration of diastole and less time available for coronary artery filling. Diastolic pressures of less than 40 mmHg are not sufficient to keep coronary blood vessels open, and pressures significantly greater than this are necessary to maintain adequate flow.

4. *Hydrostatic pressure* exerts pressure against the blood vessel wall, forcing water out. *Oncotic pressure* is the force of intravascular proteins acting to draw water into the blood vessels. These two forces *balance* each other in order to maintain equilibrium within the vascular system.

5. *Pulmonary arteries* have thinner walls and less (approximately one-sixth) *resistance* than systemic arteries, and can accommodate a three- to fourfold increase in blood volume before showing signs of increased pressure.

6. *Intracardiac pressure:* waveforms have specific characteristics for each chamber of the heart (Fig. 1–18).

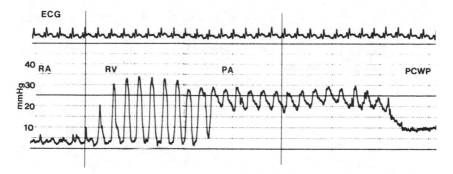

Figure 1–18. Intracardiac pressure characteristics. Tracing showing pressure waveforms seen during progression of pulmonary artery catheter from RA to RV to PA and finally wedged position (PCWP).

7. The atria have the lowest cardiac chamber pressures. *Right ventricular diastolic pressures* are approximately equal to *right atrial mean pressure. Pulmonary artery systolic and RV systolic pressures* should be equal. *PA diastolic* is higher than *RV diastolic* due to closure of the pulmonic valve.
8. *Left-sided cardiac pressure* is measured indirectly as *pulmonary capillary wedge pressures (PCWP).* PCWP reflects *left ventricular end-diastolic pressure (LVEDP),* but only during *diastole,* when the mitral valve is open. In the presence of mitral valve disease the PCWP may not be a useful reflection of LVEDP.
9. *Diastolic arterial pressure* is primarily determined by the degree of *arteriolar vasoconstriction. Pulse pressure* is primarily determined by *stroke volume and the elasticity of the aorta. Mean arterial pressure* represents the average pressure within the system during the cardiac cycle.

$$MAP = \frac{SBP + 2DBP}{3}$$

where SBP is the systolic blood pressure and DBP is the diastolic blood pressure. *Mean arterial blood pressure is* determined by *cardiac output (CO) and systemic vascular resistance (SVR):*

$$MAP = CO \times SVR$$

10. *Hemodynamic regulatory mechanisms* attempt to ensure adequate circulation to the vital organs.
11. *Cardiac output* is the product of *stroke volume and heart rate,* thus an alteration of either factor will change the cardiac output. *Heart rate changes* are the most rapid and

effective means of altering cardiac output. Stroke volume is determined by *preload* (ventricular end-diastolic pressure), *afterload* (systemic vascular resistance), and *contractility* (not clinically measurable).

12. *Systemic vascular regulation* is accomplished primarily via nervous system control. *Baroreceptors, chemoreceptors,* and the *hypothalamus* signal the *vasomotor center,* which exerts *sympathetic* effects. The venous vasculature can act as *capacitance* vessels, thus accommodating volume increases.

13. The kidneys exert a regulatory effect on the cardiovascular system via the *renin–angiotensin–aldosterone mechanism,* which serves to adjust the blood volume, thus affecting cardiac output.

Section 1 Quiz

For each multiple choice question circle the letter that corresponds to the correct answer.

1. Starling's law of the heart involves the ability of the ventricle to vary its force of contraction as a function of
   a. sympathetic tone
   b. stroke volume
   c. myocardial fiber length
   d. number of electrical impulses

2. According to Starling's law, increased ventricular volume should result in
   i. increased myocardial fiber length
   ii. increased force of contraction
   iii. increased stroke volume
   iv. increased heart rate
      a. i and ii
      b. i, ii, and iii
      c. iv only
      d. all of the above

3. Rapid transmission of impulses throughout the myocardium is possible because
   a. the cell boundaries have low impedance to electrical flow
   b. sarcomeres are composed of proteins
   c. sympathetic impulses are very strong
   d. there are norepinephrine receptors in cardiac cells

4. The autonomic nervous system regulates
   i. sensation of pain from the epicardium
   ii. formation and conduction of electrical impulses in the heart

   iii. contractility of the ventricles
   iv. vascular tone

     a. i only
     b. ii only
     c. ii, iii, and iv
     d. all of the above

5. Which of the following can affect coronary blood flow?
   i. duration of diastole
   ii. diastolic blood pressure
   iii. atherosclerosis
   iv. tachycardia

     a. i, ii, and iii
     b. ii only
     c. iii and iv
     d. all of the above

6. Increased hydrostatic pressure could cause
     a. pulmonary edema
     b. fluid overload
     c. decreased serum proteins
     d. decreased oncotic pressure

7. Decreased oncotic pressure could result from
     a. decreased serum proteins
     b. dehydration
     c. hyperglycemia
     d. decreased hydrostatic pressure

8. Pulmonary vascular resistance is lower than systemic vascular resistance because pulmonary arteries
     a. are shorter than systemic arteries
     b. receive less blood than the aorta
     c. have a thinner medial muscle layer
     d. carry unoxygenated blood

9. Decreased compliance of the ventricle in *early* diastole can result in
     a. first heart sound (S_1)
     b. second heart sound (S_2)
     c. third heart sound (S_3)
     d. fourth heart sound (S_4)

10. Right ventricular diastolic pressure is normally equal to
    a. pulmonary artery diastolic pressure
    b. pulmonary artery mean pressure
    c. left ventricular systolic pressure
    d. right atrial mean pressure

11. Right ventricular systolic pressure is normally equal to
    a. pulmonary artery systolic pressure
    b. pulmonary artery diastolic pressure
    c. right atrial mean pressure
    d. pulmonary capillary wedge pressure

12. The dicrotic notch in the PA waveform represents
    a. opening of the mitral valve
    b. closure of the tricuspid valve
    c. opening of the aortic valve
    d. closure of the pulmonic valve

13. Left ventricular end-diastolic pressure can be estimated by
    i. PCWP
    ii. PA diastolic
    iii. PA systolic
    iv. RV systolic
        a. i and ii
        b. i and iii
        c. none of above
        d. all of the above

14. Pressures obtained by occluding the pulmonary artery reflect left ventricular pressure
    a. during ventricular systole only
    b. during ventricular diastole only
    c. during both systole and diastole
    d. when the mitral valve is closed

15. Cardiac output is equal to
    a. stroke volume times heart rate
    b. mean arterial pressure times resistance
    c. PCWP times heart rate
    d. stroke volume times filling pressure

16. Increased heart rate can result in
    i. increased cardiac output
    ii. increased myocardial oxygen demands

iii. decreased coronary blood flow

iv. increased stroke volume

   a. ii

   b. i, ii, and iii

   c. i and iv

   d. all of the above

17. Stroke volume is determined by

   i. preload

   ii. afterload

   iii. contractility

   iv. total circulating blood volume

    a. i

    b. i and ii

    c. ii, iii, and iv

    d. all of the above

18. Preload is influenced by

   i. total blood volume

   ii. atrial kick

   iii. diastolic filling pressure

   iv. venous return of blood to heart

    a. i, ii, and iii

    b. i and iv

    c. ii, iii, and iv

    d. all of the above

19. Afterload refers to

   a. end-diastolic volume

   b. resistance to systolic ejection of blood

   c. left ventricular filling pressure

   d. total volume of blood in the blood vessels

20. A pharmacologic agent that increases myocardial contractility is said to have

   a. positive chronotopic effect

   b. a positive inotropic effect

   c. a negative inotropic effect

   d. a deleterious effect

21. Myocardial contractility can be decreased by

   i. hypoxemia (severe)

   ii. increased P_{CO_2}

iii. positive inotropic agent

iv. excessive fluid overload

    a. i and ii

    b. i, ii, and iv

    c. iii only

    d. all of the above

22. Systemic vascular regulation is accomplished by

    i. voluntary control

    ii. local autoregulation

    iii. vasomotor center control

    iv. autonomic nervous system control

    a. i only

    b. i and iii

    c. ii, iii, and iv

    d. all of the above

23. A patient has a blood pressure of 100/60 mmHg. His mean arterial pressure is

    a. 80 mmHg

    b. 58 mmHg

    c. 73 mmHg

    d. 40 mmHg

24. The activation of the renin–angiotensin–aldosterone mechanism

    i. results in retention of sodium and water

    ii. results from low renal blood flow

    iii. results in increased blood pressure

    iv. is an attempt to ensure adequate circulation to the vital organs

    a. i and ii

    b. ii only

    c. i, iii, and iv

    d. all of the above

25. Pulse pressure is determined by

    a. stroke volume and the elasticity of the aorta

    b. amount of arterial vasoconstriction

    c. cardiac output times systemic vascular resistance

    d. systolic pressure + 2(diastolic pressure)

Section 1 Quiz Answers

The bracketed numbers following each answer indicate the pages where discussions for each question can be found.

1. c [4]	14. b [17]
2. b [4]	15. a [21]
3. a [1]	16. b [22]
4. c [4, 25]	17. d [23]
5. d [6]	18. d [23]
6. a [8]	19. b [23]
7. a [9]	20. b [24]
8. c [7]	21. b [24]
9. c [9]	22. c [25]
10. d [14]	23. c $\dfrac{100 + 2(60)}{3} = 73$ [20]
11. a [15]	
12. d [15]	24. d [26]
13. a [17]	25. a [20]

If you had any incorrect answers, go back and review the areas you had difficulty with, then try those questions again. Once you feel that you fully understand the information presented in Section 1, proceed to Section 2.

Section 1 References

1. Berne RM, Levy MN: Cardiovascular Physiology, 4th ed. St. Louis: C. V. Mosby, 1981
2. Braunwald E, Ross J, Sonnenblick EH: Mechanisms of Contraction of the Normal and Failing Heart, 2nd ed. Boston: Little, Brown, 1976
3. Forsberg SA: Relationships between pressure in pulmonary artery, left atrium, and left ventricle with special reference to events at end diastole. Br Heart J 33:494, 1971
4. Gersher JA: Effect of positive and end-expiratory pressure on pulmonary capillary wedge pressure. Heart Lung 12(1):28, 1983
5. Grossman W, Barry WH: Diastolic pressure–volume relationships in the diseased heart. Fed Proc 39:148, 1980
6. Guyton AC: Textbook of Medical Physiology, 6th ed. Philadelphia: W. B. Saunders, 1981
7. Karliner JS, Gregoratos G: Coronary Care. New York: Churchill Livingstone, 1981
8. Kaye W: Invasive monitoring techniques. Heart Lung 12(4):408, 1983
9. King E: Influence of mechanical ventilation and pulmonary disease on pulmonary artery pressure monitoring. CMA J 121:903, 1979
10. Langfitt DE: Critical Care Certification Preparation and Review. Bowie, MD: Robert J Brady, 1984
11. Manjuran RS, Agarwal JB, Roy SB: Relationship of pulmonary artery diastolic and wedge pressure in mitral stenosis. Am Heart J 89:207, 1975
12. Mueller H, Ayres S, Giannelli S, et al: Trans NY Acad Sci Ser II 34(4):309, 1972
13. Nemens EJ, Woods SL: Normal fluctuations in pulmonary artery and pulmonary capillary wedge pressure in acutely ill patients. Heart Lung 11(5):393–398, 1982
14. Rushmer RF: Cardiovascular Dynamics. Philadelphia: W. B. Saunders, 1976
15. Sedlock S: Interpretation of hemodynamic pressures and recognition of complications. Crit Care Nurse 39, Nov–Dec 1980
16. Smiseth OA, Refsum H, Tyberg JV: Pericardial pressure assessed by right atrial pressure: A basis for calculation of left ventricular transmural pressure. Am Heart J 108(3):603, 1984

17. Starling EH: The Linacre Lecture on the Law of the Heart, Given at Cambridge, 1915. London: Longman, 1918, p. 27
18. Nij D, Babcock R, Magilligan DJ: A simplified concept of complete physiological monitoring of the critically ill patient. Heart Lung 10:75, 1981

Determination of Cardiac Output and Derived Hemodynamic Parameters

This section is an introduction to the measurement of cardiac output and to the information about ventricular performance that can be obtained through calculated hemodynamic parameters. Only those calculated parameters that can be obtained using data available at the bedside are discussed.

CARDIAC OUTPUT MEASUREMENTS

Cardiac output is the amount of blood pumped per minute from the heart. It is normally expressed in liters per minute. Cardiac output determination is extremely valuable in evaluating left ventricular function. Since cardiac output varies from person to person, depending on age, size, and overall body metabolism, serial cardiac output measurements are necessary in order to assess the patient's left ventricular function and response to treatment.

There are several methods by which cardiac output can be measured. The three most common techniques include:

- The Fick method
- The dye-dilution method
- The thermodilution method

Of these methods, the thermodilution method is the most commonly used. As this method is the one you will be exposed to most frequently, it is discussed in detail while the other two methods are briefly reviewed.

Normal resting cardiac output: *4* to *8* liters/min

Fick Method

This technique is based on Adolph Fick's principle that the uptake of oxygen by the lungs is the product of the blood flow through the lungs (CO) and the arterial–venous oxygen content difference (a-v O_2 difference). If we can determine arterial–venous oxygen difference and oxygen consumption, we can calculate cardiac output:

$$\text{Cardiac output} = \frac{O_2 \text{ consumption}}{\text{Arterial } O_2 \text{ content} - \text{Venous } O_2 \text{ content}}$$

The classic illustration of the Fick method of cardiac output determination is to imagine that the hemoglobin in the blood is represented by boxcars which pick up a load of oxygen from the alveolus in the lung and then unload part of this oxygen in the body tissues. Each of these imaginary boxcars represents 100 ml of blood, which can hold a maximum of 20 ml of oxygen (arterial O_2 content). If the boxcars return to the lungs with 15 ml of oxygen (venous O_2 content), they can each pick up 5 ml of additional oxygen in the lungs (a-v O_2 difference or a-v DO_2). If we determine that 250 ml of oxygen is taken up by the lungs every minute, and we know that each boxcar picks up 5 ml of oxygen, we can calculate the number of boxcars that must have passed through the lungs:

$$\begin{aligned}
\text{Number of "boxcars"} \atop \text{per minute} &= \frac{\text{Uptake (consumption)}}{\begin{matrix}\text{Amount of } O_2 & \text{Amount of } O_2 \\ \text{in arterial} & - \text{ in venous} \\ \text{"boxcars"} & \text{"boxcars"}\end{matrix}} \\[2mm]
&= \frac{250 \text{ ml}}{20 \text{ ml} - 15 \text{ ml}} \\[2mm]
&= \frac{250 \text{ ml}}{5 \text{ ml}} \\[2mm]
&= 50
\end{aligned}$$

Since each boxcar represents 100 ml of blood, 50 boxcars equals 50×100 ml = 5000 ml and the cardiac output equals 5000 ml (or 5 liters) per minute (Fig. 2–1).

To gather the necessary information for Fick method of cardiac output determination we need:

1. Simultaneous collection of arterial and pulmonary artery (mixed venous) blood samples for blood gas analysis. The difference in oxygen content between these samples is the *a-v O_2 difference* (a-v DO_2).

    Pulmonary artery blood is obtained from the distal port of the pulmonary artery catheter. Since venous blood from all parts of the body mixes in the right side of the heart, a

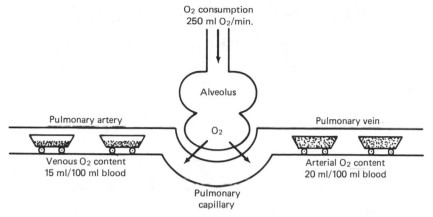

Figure 2–1. Illustration of the Fick principle. Uptake of oxygen from alveolus by boxcars (RBCs) in the pulmonary capillary.

blood sample taken from the right ventricle or pulmonary artery actually represents mixed systemic venous blood. *Mixed venous* blood samples give an accurate measurement of overall venous oxygen content whereas blood drawn from a peripheral vein reflects only the oxygen content from the particular body portion drained by that vessel.

2. Sample of expired gas from the patient and knowledge of the inspired oxygen. *Oxygen consumption* is calculated from the oxygen content of inspired gas minus oxygen content of expired gas and the patient's respiratory rate. Patient's height and weight, plus barometric pressure and temperature of the environment, are also needed to calculate oxygen consumption.

Collection of expired air and direct measurement of oxygen consumption is a cumbersome and often technically difficult procedure. Oxygen consumption can, however, be estimated by multiplying the patient's body surface area by 130 ml/min. One hundred thirty milliliters represents oxygen consumption per square meter of body surface area in the basal metabolic state.[1] However, since the oxygen consumption of individuals who are ill cannot be predicted from standardized tables, less confidence can be placed in these results.

EXAMPLE:

A patient with an acute anterior MI is admitted to the ICU. Using the following data, calculate the cardiac output, using an estimation of oxygen consumption:

Body surface area: 1.9 m^2
Arterial O_2 content: 19 ml/100 ml
Venous O_2 content: 12 ml/100 ml

$$\text{Cardiac output} = \frac{O_2 \text{ consumption}}{\text{a-v } DO_2}$$

$$= \frac{130 \text{ ml/m}^2 \times 1.9 \text{ m}^2}{19 \text{ ml/100 ml} - 12 \text{ ml/100 ml}}$$

$$= \frac{247 \text{ ml/min}}{7 \text{ ml/100 ml } or \text{ 0.07 ml}}$$

$$= 3529 \text{ ml/min or 3.53 liters/min}$$

Therefore, cardiac output by Fick estimation is 3.53 liters/min.

There are advantages and disadvantages in using the Fick method of cardiac output determination. This method is accurate, even in the presence of intracardiac shunts and valvular insufficiencies. It is a lengthy procedure, however, and requires collection of expired air and arterial and mixed venous blood for analysis. If the patient is receiving oxygen by mask or nasal prongs, it is often difficult to accurately assess inspired oxygen content, so accuracy of the cardiac output determination may be impaired. Estimation of oxygen consumption, while easier and faster, may yield an inaccurate cardiac output determination.

Dye-Dilution Method
Use of this method is usually limited to cardiac catheterization labs. (The dye-dilution method and the thermodilution method are both examples of the indicator dilution principle. See Thermodilution Method, page 43.)

The indicator in this method is a dye that is water soluble, nontoxic, and neither rapidly metabolized nor removed from the blood. This method involves the injection of a specific amount of dye into the venous circulation. Arterial blood is steadily withdrawn through a detector (densitometer) that continuously measures the concentration of dye in the blood. The concentration of dye rises rapidly to its peak height and then declines. Because the dye will recirculate, a discrete second curve may be recorded. Small, specifically designed computers measure the area under the curve and predict the decline of the first curve, thus eliminating the recirculation, and calculate cardiac output using the following formula:

$$\text{Cardiac output (liters/min)} = \frac{I \times 60}{A}$$

where

I=indicator of amount injected (mg)
60=conversion factor from seconds to minutes
A=area under the first peak of the concentration–time curve
(mg/liter × sec)

(See Fig. 2–2 for representation of indicator-dye cardiac output curve.)

This method is rapid and more easily performed than the Fick method. It is also not affected by oxygen administration. Its disadvantages include the need for venous and arterial catheters with removal of blood samples, and the requirement for an appropriate recording device and computer or tedious calculation. It is less accurate than the Fick method in the presence of low cardiac output states, intracardiac shunts, and valvular insufficiency. The presence of rapid recirculation may also decrease the accuracy of this method.

Thermodilution Method

The thermodilution technique is also based on the principle that if a known amount of indicator is added to an unknown volume of fluid and adequate time is allowed for mixing, the volume of fluid may be determined by analyzing a sample of the fluid for indicator concentration. This was also the basis for the dye-dilution method dis-

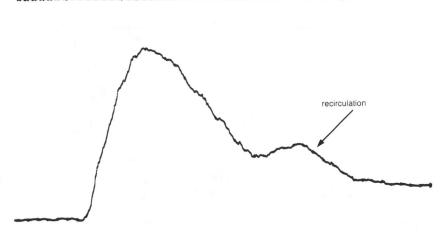

Figure 2–2. Time concentration curve using dye-dilution method of cardiac output determination. Note small second curve resulting from recirculation of dye.

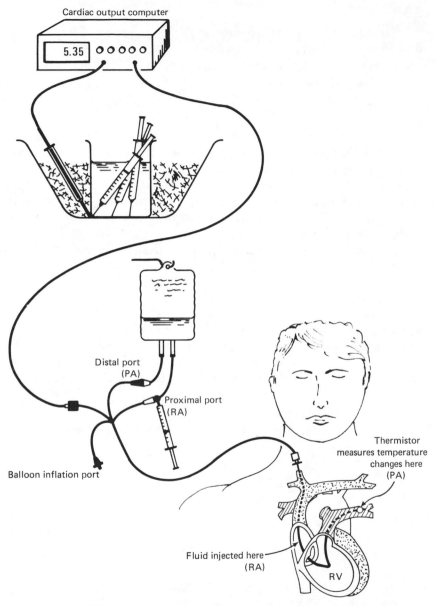

Figure 2–3. Illustration of setup and apparatus for the thermodilution method of cardiac output determination.

cussed earlier. In the thermodilution method the indicator is usually a 5% dextrose solution (D_5W) at a known temperature, different from the temperature of the blood (in common practice, always cooler).

This method requires the insertion of a thermodilution pulmo-

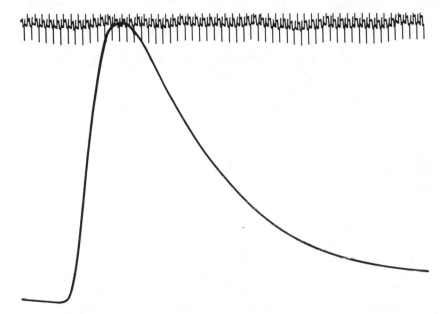

Figure 2–4. Time–temperature curve for thermodilution cardiac output determination.

nary artery catheter that has a temperature-sensing device (thermistor) on the distal tip. A small known amount of D_5W is injected into the right atrium via the proximal port of the pulmonary artery catheter. Temperature change is monitored downstream in the pulmonary artery, where the thermistor sits (Fig. 2–3).

The formula used to calculate the cardiac output by this method uses the principle that heat gain recorded when the injectate is mixed with blood is equal to heat lost by the blood. The formula is complex and requires knowledge of the following variables:

1. Volume of injectate
2. Temperature of injectate
3. Temperature of the blood
4. The area under the curve resulting from graphing temperature vs. time (Fig. 2–4)

The formula for thermodilution cardiac output determination is:

$$CO = \frac{V \times (T_B \times T_I)}{A} \times \frac{(S_I \times C_I)}{(S_B \times C_B)} \times \frac{(60 \times C_T \times K)}{} \times PS$$

where

CO	=	cardiac output (ml/min)
V	=	volume of injectate (ml)
A	=	area of thermodilution curve (mm^2)
PS	=	paper speed (mm/sec)
K	=	calibration constant (mm/°C)
T_B, T_I	=	temperature of blood (B) and injectate (I)
S_B, S_I	=	specific gravity of blood (B) and injectate (I)
C_B, C_I	=	specific heat of blood (B) and injectate (I)
$\dfrac{(S_I \times C_I)}{(S_B \times C_B)}$	=	1.08 when 5% dextrose is used
60	=	60 sec/min
C_T	=	correction factor for injectate warming

A cardiac output computer is connected to the thermistor outlet on the pulmonary artery catheter and calculates cardiac output from this information. It is important that the amount of D_5W drawn up into the syringes be exact and that the temperature of the injectate be carefully monitored. If iced injectate is used, a temperature registering device is placed in the ice bath with syringes of injectate. The device should not touch the side of the ice bath container, especially if the container is metal, as this can give an inaccurate temperature reading. To ensure that the temperature registered by the probe is the same as the injectate temperature, it is suggested that the probe be inserted into an capped syringe barrel filled with injectate and then into the ice bath. To keep the temperature of the D_5W from decreasing significantly, it is important that the syringes not be removed from the ice bath until immediately before injection and that syringes not be handled excessively or held by the barrel. The injectate should be injected rapidly and smoothly in the proximal port of the pulmonary artery catheter to ensure uniform mixing of the D_5W with the venous return.

The accuracy of this method depends on careful technique in measurement of injectate, rapidity and consistency of injection (less than 10 seconds should elapse from removal of syringe from ice bath to completion of injection), and in timing each injection so that it occurs during the same phase of respiration. Since venous return to the heart changes during respiration (due to changes in intrathoracic pressure), timing the injection to coincide with the same phase of respiration helps maintain consistency. *End expiration* is the preferred phase in which to inject the D_5W. To ensure a representative cardiac output measurement, it is suggested that at least three injections be carried out. These three measurements are then averaged to give the actual cardiac output determination. Each of the cardiac output measurements should be within 10% of each other. If greater variation occurs between the serial measurements it could reflect either poor or inconsistent technique. There are instances, however, when inconsistent serial determinations may reflect true changes in cardiac output. These changes may be due to any of the following:

1. Variations in cardiac rate or rhythm, e.g., premature ventricular contractions (PVCs). (Keep an eye on the ECG monitor so that such an occurrence is not missed.)
2. Patient movement, which may alter venous return to the heart and thus change cardiac output.
3. A change in injectate temperature.
4. A drastic change in patient temperature.
5. A sudden change in hemodynamic state of the patient.
6. The presence of valvular insufficiency or intracardiac shunt. (These conditions make cardiac output measurement by this technique inaccurate and unreliable.)

There are several advantages to the thermodilution method of cardiac output determination, and for these reasons it is the most commonly used method of bedside cardiac output measurement. Only one catheter is required, and this pulmonary artery catheter can be inserted at the bedside. In fact, the patient who requires cardiac output measurement is likely to have a pulmonary artery catheter in place already, and if the catheter is equipped for thermodilution, no further invasive procedures are necessary. Blood withdrawal is not required, serial determinations can be performed rapidly (within 60 seconds), and reproducibility is good provided injection technique is consistent. The results are not affected by oxygen administration and a second recirculation peak is very seldom a problem. It is generally a simple, easily performed technique.

The disadvantages of this technique include potential electrical hazards should thermistor wires become damaged, as well as the possible hazards of an indwelling pulmonary artery catheter. Fluid overloading the patient is a potential problem if numerous and frequent determinations are performed. The potential for contamination of injectate and introduction of infection also exists. There have been reports of transient bradycardia and atrial fibrillation occurring with use of iced injectate.[10,14] This technique will be somewhat less accurate in low cardiac output states (although it is more accurate than the dye-dilution technique) and is definitely not accurate in the presence of intracardiac shunts or valvular insufficiency.[2]

The thermodilution method is actually determining *right* ventricular cardiac output. Despite the gross differences in the shape, wall thickness, and outflow resistance of the right and left ventricles, they of course must eject the same amount of blood averaged over any significant period of time. If right ventricular cardiac output exceeded left ventricular output, the lungs would become congested with blood while the systemic vasculatures would be depleted. Thus there is equalization of right and left cardiac outputs, and by using the thermodilution technique we are indirectly measuring left ventricular cardiac output. This assumes, of course, that no intracardiac shunts are present.

Procedure

The thermodilution technique is the most commonly used method for bedside determination of cardiac output, and consistent, careful technique is important in order to ensure reliable results. For these reasons a brief review of procedure is indicated. This review is generalized and is intended to stress the procedural principles that are important regardless of the exact type or model of cardiac output computer used.

1. Ensure that the patient has a thermodilution-equipped pulmonary artery catheter in the proper position, as validated by waveform analysis and x-rays.
2. Fill syringes (all the same size) with *exact* amount of sterile D_5W. Specific unit policies may vary. Some units use 5 ml of injectate and others use 10 ml. It is important, however, that you use the amount specified by the type of equipment you are using and the computation constant programmed into your cardiac output computer. Cap syringes with covered needles. Sterility of the D_5W must be maintained, as it will be injected into the patient. One way to ensure sterility is to place the syringes in a 500-ml sterile beaker filled with sterile saline, or use a closed system (Fig. 2–5A,B).
3. Prepare an ice bath. Ice and water is a more effective cooling system than is ice alone, since a slush solution provides greater surface area for cooling around the syringe or beaker.
4. Place beaker full of syringes and saline in the ice bath for

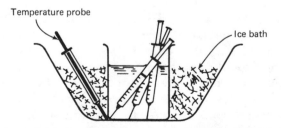

Figure 2–5A. Setup of syringes in ice bath to maintain sterility of injectate during thermodilution method cardiac output determination.

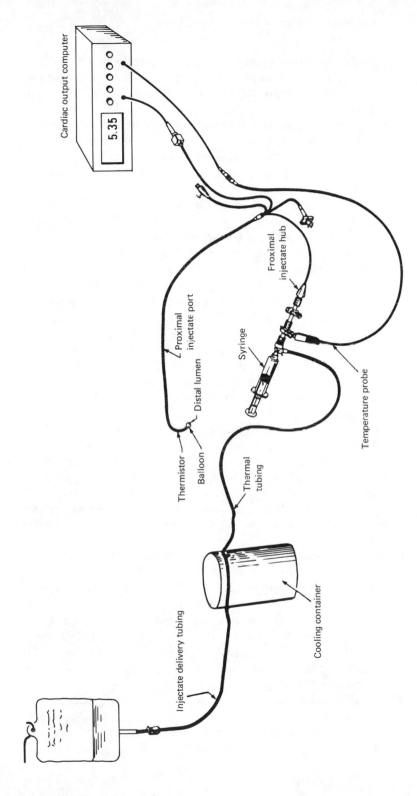

Figure 2–5B. Alternate setup for thermodilution cardiac output determination using a closed system.

49

at least 45 minutes (preferably longer) before use. This length of time is necessary for complete cooling of injectate. Incomplete or uneven cooling will result in inaccurate results.

5. Place the temperature-monitoring device from the cardiac output computer into the capped barrel of a syringe of injectate. Place the device and syringe barrel into the ice bath.

6. Plug in cardiac output computer and turn it on. Level and calibrate transducer.

7. Record patient's heart rate, pulmonary artery systolic, diastolic, mean, and wedge pressures, mean right atrial pressure ($\overline{\text{RA}}$), and mean arterial pressure (MAP):

8. Calibrate the cardiac output computer as per instructions on the machine. This calibration procedure should not be carried out more than 15 minutes before performing the actual cardiac output determinations. Ensure that your cardiac output computer is calibrated to the type of pulmonary artery catheter you are using. Pulmonary artery (PA) catheters with extra venous infusion ports have a different computation constant than do regular PA catheters. The information concerning exact constants should be included with the cardiac output computer and/or PA catheter package insert.

9. Ensure that the proximal port of the pulmonary artery catheter is not being used to administer continuous drip medications. If so, move the IV to another site. Withdraw on the proximal line to clear the medication and prevent inadvertent bolus administration with injecting the D_5W.

10. Ensure that the start button or pedal is close beside you as you stand ready to perform the cardiac output determination.

11. Take a syringe from the ice bath, remove the needle, and insert the syringe into the stopcock on the proximal port of the pulmonary artery catheter. Turn the stopcock open to the proximal port and rapidly and smoothly inject the D_5W during the end-expiration phase of the patient's respiratory cycle, pressing the "Start" device as you begin injecting.

12. Turn the stopcock off to the syringe upon completion of the injection. Discard the syringe. Make sure to avoid contaminating the stopcock port.

13. Record cardiac output as it appears on the digital display on the computer.

14. When "RDY" appears on the face of the digital display, you may repeat steps 11 through 13.

Three to five serial injections should be done, depending on your unit policy. When five injections are done, often 5 ml injections are used to limit amount of fluid given. If five injections are performed, usually the highest and lowest of these are rejected and the remaining three are averaged to give the cardiac output measurement. If only three are done, all three are averaged. It is recommended that the type and amount of vasoactive drugs being administered be noted and included with the results of the cardiac output determinations.

Variations in Procedure

In some centers room-temperature injectate is used instead of iced injectate. Iced injectate has been said to reduce the variability in cardiac output due to respiration-induced pulmonary artery temperature changes, so-called *physiologic noise*. It was believed that the increased signal-to-noise ratio that results from using iced injectate ensures more accurate cardiac output determinations. Recent studies have found that room-temperature injectate results compared favorably with those obtained using iced injectate, and there may be advantages in using room-temperature injectate: reduced time and expense involved in setup, reduced chance of cold-induced arrhythmias, and no need to wait while injectate cools.[7,15]

Studies have been undertaken to ascertain whether or not the volume of injectate used has any effect on the accuracy of the results. In general, either 10- or 5-ml volumes are acceptable as long as the identical volume is injected every time.[13] Use of 5-ml injectate reduces the possibility of fluid overloading susceptible patients.

Automatic injection using a CO_2 injecting gun is an alternative to the manual injection technique. Studies indicate that there are no significant differences between values obtained by the manual and automatic techniques.[9]

Injecting at the same point during the respiratory cycle (usually at end expiration phase) reduces the variability of cardiac output results. It has been suggested, however, that this does not accurately represent the average cardiac output and that thermodilution determined cardiac output is more representative of true patient status when values are obtained at regularly spaced intervals through the ventilation cycle, especially when the patient is mechanically ventilated.[6,12]

CARDIAC CALCULATIONS

The major objective of hemodynamic monitoring is to evaluate the performance of the heart as a pump. A number of hemodynamic

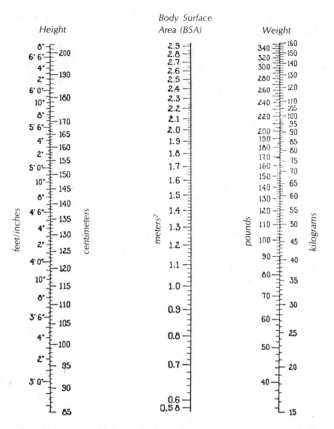

Height

Body Surface Area (BSA)

Weight

Figure 2–6. Dubois Body Surface Area chart. Find the patient's height in the left column and weight in the right column. Connect these two points with a straight line. Patient's BSA is indicated at the point where the straight line intersects the middle column.

parameters can be calculated from the pressure data and cardiac output determinations obtained through the use of the pulmonary artery catheter. These derived hemodynamic parameters serve as a basis for further evaluation of cardiac performance.

Cardiac Index

Cardiac output varies from person to person, depending on specific variables, a major variable being body size. A cardiac output of 4 liters/min might be considered normal for a petite woman, but could be inadequate for a large man. For this reason, cardiac output data are often normalized so that data among patients of varying body size can be compared. This is accomplished by dividing the cardiac output by the patient's body surface area (BSA). Body surface area is determined by the use of a nomogram. The patient's height and weight are plotted on the nomogram and a line is drawn connecting the two plotted points. The point where this line intersects the BSA line corresponds with the patient's body surface area. (Fig. 2–6).

Cardiac output normalized in this way is referred to as the cardiac index (CI). Other hemodynamic parameters, such as stroke volume and stroke work, can be similarly standardized by dividing them by the patient's BSA. These are then referred to as stroke volume index and stroke work index.

Normal CI: 2.7 to 4.3 liters/min/m²

CI values between 1.8 and 2.2 liters/min/m² indicate the onset of clinical hypoperfusion. CI values below 1.8 liters/min/m² may be associated with cardiogenic shock.[4]

Stroke Volume
Stroke volume (SV) was reviewed in Section 1 in the subsection on Cardiac Regulation (page 21). Since cardiac output equals stroke volume times heart rate, cardiac output divided by heart rate will give stroke volume:

$$CO = SV \times HR$$

$$SV = \frac{CO}{HR}$$

Normal SV: 60 to 130 ml
Normal SV index (SVI): 35 to 65 ml/m²

If a patient had a cardiac output of 5.0 liters/min and a heart rate of 100 beats/min, the stroke volume would be

$$SV = \frac{5.0 \text{ liters/min}}{100 \text{ beats/min}}$$

$$= \frac{0.05 \text{ liters}}{\text{or } 50 \text{ ml}}$$

If this patient had a BSA of 1.80 m², the stroke volume index would be

$$SVI = \frac{50 \text{ ml}}{1.80 \text{ m}^2}$$

$$= 27.8 \text{ ml/m}^2$$

Systemic Vascular Resistance
Systemic vascular resistance (also called peripheral vascular resistance) is a measure of peripheral blood vessel resistance to blood

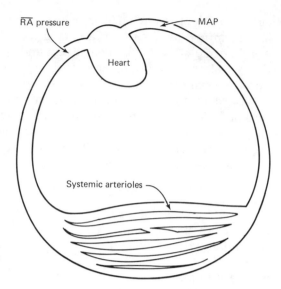

Figure 2–7. Schematic representation of systemic vascular resistance.

flow. The arterioles are the major determinants of this resistance. Resistance to flow is also referred to as afterload; therefore, in determining systemic vascular resistance (SVR) we are actually determining afterload.

To calculate SVR we need to know the patient's mean arterial pressure, $\overline{\text{RA}}$ pressure, and cardiac output values. SVR is the ratio of the pressure drop across the systemic vascular system to the total flow passing through the systemic circulation. The pressure drop can be calculated by measuring the mean pressure of blood leaving the left ventricle and entering the systemic circulation (MAP) and subtracting the mean pressure of blood leaving the systemic circulation and entering the right atrium ($\overline{\text{RA}}$ pressure) (Fig. 2–7). The total flow passing through the systemic circulation is measured as the cardiac output. So, by using measured hemodynamic parameters we can derive SVR by the following formula:

$$\text{SVR} = \frac{(\text{MAP} - \overline{\text{RA}})}{\text{CO liters/min}} \quad \text{(all pressures expressed in mmHg)}$$

It is customary in many centers to multiply the result by 80 to convert mmHg/min/liter to dynes/sec/cm^5, known as absolute resistance units. Thus the formula for calculating systemic vascular resistance is:

$$\text{SVR} = \frac{(\text{MAP} - \overline{\text{RA}}) \times 80}{\text{CO liters/min}} \quad \text{(all pressures expressed in mmHg)}$$

Note that if $\overline{\text{RA}}$ pressure is not available, it is possible to obtain a reasonable assessment of SVR without including $\overline{\text{RA}}$ *if* there is a reasonable assurance that the $\overline{\text{RA}}$ pressure is normal (i.e., 0 to 6 mmHg).

Normal SVR: *1000* to *1300* dynes/sec/cm^5

An abnormally high SVR would indicate peripheral vaso-constriction, such as might occur in response to hypovolemia. An abnormally low SVR would indicate peripheral vasodilation, as might occur in septic shock.

EXAMPLE 1:
If a patient had the following hemodynamic parameters, what would the SVR be?

$$\overline{\text{RA}}:\quad 10 \text{ mmHg}$$
$$\text{MAP}:\quad 80 \text{ mmHg}$$
$$\text{CO}:\quad 5.0 \text{ liters/min}$$
$$\text{SVR} = \frac{(80 - 10) \times 80}{5.0}$$
$$= \frac{5600}{5.0}$$

Answer: 1120 dynes/sec/cm^5

EXAMPLE 2:
What about the patient with the following parameters?

$$\overline{\text{RA}}:\quad 14 \text{ mmHg}$$
$$\text{BP}:\quad 100/60 \text{ mmHg}$$
$$\text{CO}:\quad 4.0 \text{ liters/min}$$
$$\text{MAP} = \frac{100 + 2(60)}{3}$$
$$= 73 \text{ mmHg}$$
$$\text{SVR} = \frac{(73 - 14) \times 80}{4.0}$$
$$= \frac{4720}{4.0}$$

Answer: 1180 dynes/sec/cm^5 (within normal limits)

Pulmonary Vascular Resistance
Pulmonary vascular resistance (PVR) is sometimes referred to as *pulmonary arteriolar resistance*. It is a measure of the pulmonary blood vessel resistance to blood flow. PVR is calculated based on the same principle used to calculate SVR. PVR, then, is the ratio of the pressure drop across the pulmonary vascular system to the total flow passing through the pulmonary circulation. The pressure drop is calculated by measuring the mean pressure of blood entering the pulmonary artery ($\overline{\text{PA}}$ pressure) and subtracting the mean pressure of blood leaving the pulmonary veins (PCWP) (Fig. 2–8). The total

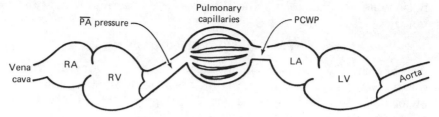

Figure 2–8. Schematic representation of pulmonary vascular resistance.

flow passing through the pulmonary circulation is measured as cardiac output. Again, it is often customary to multiply the result by 80 to convert SVR to absolute resistance units. The formula for determining PVR is therefore

$$PVR = \frac{(\overline{PA} - PCWP) \times 80}{CO} \text{ dynes/sec/cm}^5$$

Normal PVR: *150* to *250* dynes/sec/cm^5

You will note that normal PVR is approximately one sixth of the normal SVR. This was mentioned in Section 1 under Pulmonary Circulation. Refer to page 7 to review the reason for this lower resistance. An abnormally high PVR could be indicative of pulmonary hypertension, hypoxia, lung disease, or pulmonary embolism.

EXAMPLE:
If a patient has the following parameters, what is his PVR?

$$\overline{PA}: \quad 25 \text{ mmHg}$$
$$PCWP: \quad 8 \text{ mmHg}$$
$$CO: \quad 5.0 \text{ liters/min}$$
$$PVR = \frac{(25 - 8) \times 80}{5.0}$$
$$= \frac{1360}{5.0}$$

Answer: 272 dynes/sec/cm^5

Stroke Work
Stroke work (SW) is a measure of how hard the heart muscle must work to pump blood. Stroke work is determined by the average pressure generated by ventricular contraction multiplied by the amount of blood ejected by the contraction. It is affected by myocardial mass, oxygenation, preload, afterload, HR, and contractility.[16]

Right Ventricular Stroke Work
The average pressure generated by right ventricular contraction is the *pulmonary artery systolic* (PA_{sys}) pressure minus the *right atrial*

mean pressure. The $\overline{\text{RA}}$ is subtracted from the PA_{sys} because the $\overline{\text{RA}}$ represents the pressure already present in the right ventricle before contraction [remember that central venous pressure equals mean right atrial pressure equals right ventricular end-diastolic pressure (CVP-$\overline{\text{RA}}$-RVEDP)]. The amount of blood ejected by the right ventricle is the same as that ejected by the left ventricle: the *stroke volume.*

Thus the formula for determining right ventricular stroke work (RVSW) is:

$$\text{RVSW} = (\text{PA}_{\text{sys}} - \overline{\text{RA}}) \times \text{SV} \times 0.0136$$

(0.0136 is a conversion factor from millimeters of mercury per milliliter to gram-meters.)

Normal RVSW: *10* to *15* g-m/beat
Normal RVSWI: *5* to *10* g-m/beat/m^2

Left Ventricular Stroke Work

The average pressure generated by left ventricular contraction is *systolic arterial pressure* minus *PCWP* [remember that pulmonary capillary wedge pressure equals mean left atrial pressure equals left ventricular end-diastolic pressure (PCWP=$\overline{\text{LA}}$=LVEDP)]. By substituting this into the formula for RVSW, we generate the formula for left ventricular stroke work (LVSW):

$$\text{LVSW} = (\text{BP}_{\text{sys}} - \text{PCWP}) \times \text{SV} \times 0.0136$$

Normal LVSW: *60* to *80* g-m/beat
Normal LVSWI: *30* to *50* g-m/beat/m^2

EXAMPLE 1:

Calculate the RVSW and LVSW for the patient with the following hemodynamic parameters:

$\overline{\text{RA}}$:   4 mmHg
PA_{sys}: 26 mmHg
PCWP: 6 mmHg
BP: 90/70 mmHg
SV: 45 ml
RVSW $= (26 - 4) \times 45 \times 0.0136$
LVSW $= (90 - 6) \times 45 \times 0.0136$

Answer: RVSW $=$ 13.5 g-m/beat
LVSW $=$ 51.4 g-m/beat

EXAMPLE 2:

Calculate the SV, MAP, RVSW, and LVSW for this patient:

$\overline{\text{RA}}$:   4 mmHg
PA_{sys}: 23 mmHg

PCWP: 10 mmHg
BP: 110/75 mmHg
CO: 4.5 liter/min
HR: 75 beats/min

Answer: SV   = 0.060 liters, or 60 ml
MAP = 87 mmHg
RVSW = 15.5 g-m/beat
LVSW = 81.6 g-m/beat

As mentioned previously, the stroke work values can be standardized by dividing by the patient's body surface area to give stroke work index.

It is not necessary to memorize these formulas, but it is important to know how these values are obtained and what they mean. Although one determination of the patient's stroke work may not mean very much, serial determinations can demonstrate trends and indicate the effect of therapy. By assessing the patient's stroke work values, you can evaluate the performance of his or her ventricles and, in conjunction with other hemodynamic parameters, assess overall cardiac function.

Ventricular Function Curves

Invasive hemodynamic monitoring permits evaluation of the heart as a pump. By extrapolation of Starling's law of the heart, clinical assessment of hemodynamic status can be obtained. Such an assessment relates the systolic performance of left ventricular cardiac muscle to diastolic fiber length or stretch of that muscle to give a *left ventricular function curve*. Left ventricular end-diastolic pressure (LVEDP), measured as pulmonary capillary wedge pressure (PCWP), is used as the index of myocardial diastolic fiber length. Systolic performance may be measured in terms of a number of parameters:

1. Cardiac output (CO)
2. Cardiac index (CI)
3. Stroke volume (SV)
4. Stroke volume index (SVI)
5. Left ventricular stroke work (LVSW)
6. Left ventricular stroke work index (LVSWI)

Although all of the parameters listed above are indices of ventricular performance and can be used in the construction of ventricular function curves, the use of LVSW or LVSWI has an advantage. Ventricular function curves using CO or SV parameters can be shifted by changes in afterload as well as by changes in contractility. If LVSW is used, afterload will not tend to have an effect on the curve, and any shift that occurs can be attributed to a change in contractility. The reason that LVSW is less affected by afterload changes than are parameters such as CO and SV can be explained by referring to a simplified formula for calculating LVSW:

$$\text{LVSW} = \text{BP}_{\text{sys}} \times \text{SV}$$

An increase in afterload results in a decrease in stroke volume, but it also causes an elevation in systolic arterial pressure, so that the effects in essence cancel each other out.

Therefore, although any one of these parameters can be used as a measure of systolic performance, further discussion and examples are confined to left ventricular function curves obtained by plotting LVSWI against PCWP.

Most of the time, we are concerned with assessing the function of the left ventricle, but occasionally it may be important to assess the function of the right ventricle, for instance in cases of right ventricular myocardial infarction. The ventricular function curves discussed so far have been concerned with the assessment of left ventricular function. A right ventricular function curve can be obtained by plotting a measure of right ventricular systolic performance against right ventricular end-diastolic pressure (RVEDP). RVEDP is measured as $\overline{\text{RA}}$ pressure. Right ventricular systolic performance can be measured in the same fashion as any of the parameters used for left ventricular systolic performance, except that right ventricular stroke work and stroke work index are used instead of the corresponding left ventricular values.

Ventricular function curves are most useful if evaluated serially. Ongoing determinations of the patient's ventricular function curves not only helps in the assessment of the patient's initial hemodynamic status, but also evaluates the patient's response to therapeutic intervention or change in cardiovascular status.

As can be seen in Figure 2–9, the ventricular function curve can be either normal, augmented (shifted upward), or depressed (shifted downward). Upward shift of the curve is caused by increased contractility. The ventricular function curve shifts downward in response to decreased contractility. (If SV or CO are used in the ventricular function curve, decreased afterload will shift the curve upward while increased afterload will shift the curve downward.)

Just as cardiac output varies among patients, ventricular function curves also vary. By determining each patient's ventricular function curve, each patient's optimum PCWP can be determined and the optimum ventricular function level can be maintained by adjusting fluid, and vasoactive and inotropic drug administration accordingly.

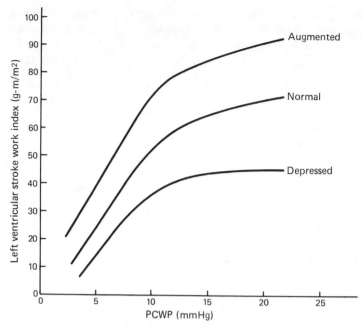

Figure 2–9. Ventricular function curve showing normal curve, augmented curve due to increased contractility, and depressed curve due to decreased contractility (failing heart). Note that a failing heart can produce less work than normal at a given filling pressure.

EXAMPLE 1:

A patient has the following hemodynamic parameters measured over the last 48 hours:

Measurement #	1	2	3	4
LVSWI	30	50	65	65
PCWP	5	10	20	25

These values are plotted on a graph (Fig. 2–10) to determine this patient's ventricular function curve. This patient's ventricular function curve is within the normal range.

EXAMPLE 2:

The data for this patient are plotted on the same graph (Fig. 2–10) to determine his ventricular function curve:

Measurement #	1	2	3	4
LVSWI	20	27	30	25
PCWP	10	15	20	25

This patient has a depressed ventricular function curve. By looking at the curve, you can see that his best LVSWI value

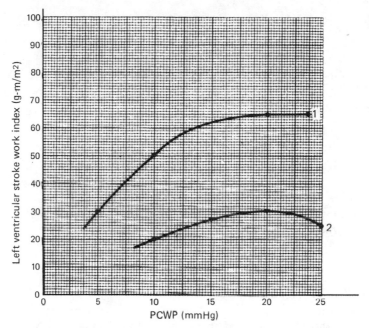

Figure 2–10. Ventricular function curves for Examples 1 and 2.

occurs when his PCWP is 18 to 22 mmHg. This range of PCWP can be maintained in an attempt to optimize this patient's ventricular performance. As mentioned earlier, depressed curves are the result of decreased contractility. Treatment aimed at enhancing contractility can help shift this patient's curve upwards, and afterload reduction can increase stroke volume, thus improving ventricular performance.

Coronary Perfusion Pressure
As mentioned in Section 1, perfusion of the coronary arteries occurs mainly during diastole, and coronary perfusion pressures less than 40 mmHg are inadequate to keep the coronary arteries open.

Since coronary blood flow occurs during diastole, and mean arterial pressure (MAP) closely represents diastolic pressure, we can estimate coronary blood flow using MAP. A formula for quick estimation of coronary artery perfusion pressures (CAPP) is:

$$CAPP = MAP - PCWP$$
Normal CAPP: *60* to *80* mmHg

- CAPP greater than 80 mmHg can result in increased resistance to flow in the coronary arteries due to reflex coronary artery vasoconstriction.
- CAPP less than 60 mmHg may be inadequate to maintain myocardial perfusion.

- CAPP less than 40 mmHg results in collapse of coronary arteries.

When checking your patient's MAP, keep in mind that even in the face of seemingly adequate MAP, if the patient has a high PCWP, he or she may not have adequate coronary artery perfusion pressures.

EXAMPLE:
A patient is admitted to the CCU with an acute anterior MI. His MAP is 70 mmHg and PCWP is 25 mmHg. His CAPP is

$$70 \text{ mmHg} - 25 \text{ mmHg} = 45 \text{ mmHg}$$

and is probably not adequate to meet myocardial tissue needs, especially in the presence of increased HR, or myocardial infarction.

MIXED VENOUS BLOOD SAMPLING

Blood samples obtained from the pulmonary artery via the distal port of the pulmonary artery catheter allow measurement of mixed venous oxygen content. By comparing this value with that of a simultaneously drawn arterial sample, the arterial–venous difference in oxygen content (as reviewed in the section on Fick cardiac output determination) can be determined. This is an indirect hemodynamic parameter; the difference in oxygen content between the arterial and mixed venous sample indicates how much oxygen has been extracted from the blood by the tissues, and this can tell us something about the cardiac output. When cardiac output is reduced, e.g., in hypovolemic shock, blood remains in the capillaries for a relatively long time, allowing greater extraction of oxygen by the tissues, which results in a lowered oxygen content in the mixed venous sample, and a larger arterial–venous oxygen content difference (a-v DO_2).

On the other hand, when cardiac output is increased, e.g., in septic shock, blood remains in the capillaries for a relatively short time and may even be shunted past capillary beds. This would result in less oxygen being removed from the blood, and mixed venous oxygen content would be closer to the arterial oxygen content and a-v DO_2 would be decreased.

Normal a-v DO_2: *4* to *6* vol.%

- Increased a-v DO_2 indicates decreased cardiac output
- Decreased a-v DO_2 indicates increased cardiac output

NOTE: We are assuming that all other factors affecting arterial oxygenation are normal.

In order to obtain accurate mixed venous oxygen content values, proper techniques in drawing the pulmonary artery sample must be followed.[11] The balloon must be deflated and the PA catheter must not be in a wedged position. The distal port of the PA catheter should be registering an adequate PA waveform. Blood must be withdrawn slowly to ensure that blood is not pulled back from alveolar capillaries. These precautions are taken to ensure that arterialized blood is not obtained. Arterialized blood has a higher Po_2 and lower Pco_2 than does mixed venous blood. To ensure that arterialized blood has not been inadvertently drawn from the PA distal port, a sample of simultaneously drawn systemic arterial blood can be compared to the mixed venous sample. If the Pco_2 of the blood drawn from the PA catheter is not at least 2 mmHg greater than the Pco_2 of the systemic arterial sample, it is likely that arterialized blood has been obtained instead of mixed venous blood.

Arterial and mixed venous oxygenation can also be determined by analyzing the *oxygen saturation* of the red blood cells. Oxygen saturation measures the extent to which the hemoglobin of the red blood cells is filled to capacity with oxygen and is recorded as a percentage. It is conventionally measured using spectrophotometric techniques that depend on precise evaluation of the hemoglobin's change in color (from reddish blue to red) as more and more oxygen is added to the blood.

> Normal arterial O_2 saturation: *95%*
> Mixed venous O_2 saturation: *70 to 75%*

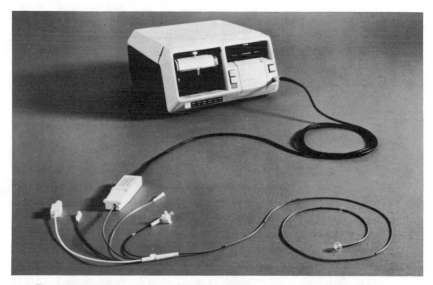

Figure 2–11. Opticath fiber optic pulmonary artery catheter for continuous monitoring of mixed venous oxygen saturation. *(With permission of Oximetrix, Inc.)*

Mixed venous oxygen saturation can be monitored through the use of a fiberoptic pulmonary artery catheter that permits continous monitoring of mixed venous oxygen saturation and allows determination of the standard hemodynamic measurements, including thermodilution cardiac outputs.[3] The fiberoptic catheter method is a special spectrophotometric technique adapted to allow intravascular measurements of oxygen saturation. The fiberoptic channel in this catheter emits a pulsatile red light from the catheter tip into the pulmonary artery. The wavelength of this reflected light depends on the color of the hemoglobin in the red blood cells and, thus, their oxygen saturation. The reflected light is conducted to a photodetector and to a computer that measures the light intensity at selected wavelengths and calculates oxygen saturation.

Continuous monitoring of mixed venous oxygen can be valuable for detecting deterioration in the patient's cardiopulmonary status and for monitoring the effect of therapeutic intervention (Fig. 2–11).

Summary of Important Concepts in Section 2

1. *Cardiac output* is the amount of blood pumped per minute by the heart (in liters per minute). The most common method of determining cardiac output is the *thermodilution method*. There are advantages and disadvantages in using each of the three major techniques of cardiac output determination:

Method	Advantages	Disadvantages
Fick method	Accurate in presence of intracardiac shunts and valvular disease Gives an indication of patient's respiratory status	Lengthy, complicated procedure Requires collection of expired air and arterial and mixed venous blood Inaccurate in presence of oxygen per mask or nasal prongs
Dye method	Rapidly performed Not affected by oxygen administration	Less accurate in presence of low-cardiac-output states, intracardiac shunts, and valvular insufficiency Requires administration of dye to patient and insertion of two catheters (arterial and venous) Results affected by rapid recirculation
Thermodilution method	Need for only one catheter No blood withdrawal necessary Rapid and reproducible Not affected by oxygen administration Simple and easily performed	Potential electrical hazard Less accurate in low-cardiac-output states, intracardiac shunts, and valvular disease

Cardiac output can be standardized in relation to body size by dividing it by body surface area to give *cardiac index*. Other hemodynamic parameters can also be standardized by dividing them by BSA, and they are then referred to as an *index* of that parameter.

2. *Formulas* for calculated hemodynamic parameters:

Parameter	Formula	Normal Values
Cardiac output	$CO = HR \times SV$	4–8 liters/min
Cardiac index	$CI = CO \div BSA$	2.7–4.3 liters/min/m²
Stroke volume	$SV = CO \div HR$	60–130 ml
Stroke volume index	$SVI = SV \div BSA$	35–65 ml/m²
Systemic vascular resistance	$SVR = \dfrac{(MAP - \overline{RA})80}{CO}$	1000–1300 dynes/sec/cm⁵
Pulmonary vascular resistance	$PVR = \dfrac{(\overline{PA} - PCWP)80}{CO}$	150–250 dynes/sec/cm⁵
Left ventricular stroke work	$LVSW = (BP_{sys} - PCWP) \times SV \times 0.0136$	60–80 g-m/beat
Left ventricular stroke work index	$LVSWI = LVSW \div BSA$	30–50 g-m/beat/m²
Right ventricular stroke work	$RVSW = (PA_{sys} - \overline{RA}) \times SV \times 0.0136$	10–15 g-m/beat
Right ventricular stroke work index	$RVSWI = RVSW \div BSA$	5–10 g-m/beat/m²
Coronary artery perfusion pressure	$CAPP = MAP - PCWP$	60–80 mmHg
Arterial–venous oxygen difference	a-v DO₂ = Arterial O₂ content − Mixed venous O₂ content	4–6 vol.%

3. *Ventricular function curves* relate parameters of systolic performance such as cardiac index, stroke work index, or stroke volume index to measurements of myocardial fiber stretch as assessed by PCWP (left ventricular preload). An *upward shift* of the curve can occur in response to

- Increased contractility
- Decreased afterload (except when stroke work is used)

A *downward shift* of the ventricular function curve can occur in response to

- Decreased contractility
- Increased afterload (except when stroke work is used)

By determining the patient's ventricular function curve, you can determine each patient's *optimum PCWP* (and therefore preload), and this optimum level can be maintained by adjusting fluid, vasoactive, and inotropic drug administration accordingly. The patient's curve can be shifted downward or upward by altering contractility.

4. *Right ventricular function curves* can be obtained using parameters of right ventricular systolic performance, such as cardiac index, or right ventricular stroke work index plotted against RA pressure. This would be useful in assessing right ventricular function in the presence of right ventricular myocardial infarction.

5. *Mixed venous blood sampling* can be used as an indirect hemodynamic parameter. It can alert us to changes in cardiac output when mixed venous oxygen content and the oxygen content of simultaneously drawn systemic arterial blood are compared. Continuous monitoring of mixed venous oxygen saturation gives the same information and can be accomplished through the use of a fiberoptic pulmonary artery catheter.

Section 2 Quiz

For each multiple choice question circle the letter that corresponds to the correct answer. For each short answer question fill in the answer in the space provided.

1. The advantages of the Fick cardiac output method are:
    i. accuracy in the presence of intracardiac shunts
    ii. accuracy in the presence of mitral insufficiency
    iii. it is rapidly and easily performed
    iv. it is not affected by oxygen administration
    v. it gives an indication of the patient's respiratory status

    a. iii only
    b. i and ii
    c. i, ii, and v
    d. all of the above

2. The accuracy of the dye-dilution cardiac output method is decreased by:
    i. rapid recirculation of dye
    ii. presence of intracardiac shunts
    iii. presence of low-cardiac-output states
    iv. presence of valvular insufficiency
    v. administration of oxygen by mask

    a. i only
    b. ii and iv
    c. i, ii, iii, and iv
    d. all of the above

3. Which of the following is true regarding the Fick method of cardiac output determination?
    a. Oxygen consumption is divided by a-v DO_2.
    b. It requires the injection of dye into the pulmonary artery.

c. It is totally noninvasive.

d. It requires the patient to be unconscious.

4. The thermodilution cardiac output method requires knowledge of:

   i. volume of injectate

   ii. temperature of injectate

   iii. temperature of patient's blood

   iv. oxygen consumption

   v. oxygen content

     a. ii and iii

     b. i, ii, and iii

     c. iv and v

     d. all of the above

5. When performing thermodilution cardiac output determinations, it is important to:

   i. maintain sterility of the iced D_5W

   ii. measure the volume of injectate accurately

   iii. make sure less than 10 seconds elapse between removing syringe from ice bath and completion of injection

   iv. time the injections to occur during end expiration

   v. make sure injections are done smoothly and consistently

     a. i and ii

     b. iv only

     c. i, ii, iii, and v

     d. all of the above

6. The following five cardiac output measurements were done serially. The cardiac output value that would be recorded is:

     4.8   5.9   5.3   5.5   5.6

7. Inconsistent serial cardiac output determinations (thermodilution method) could reflect:

   i. poor or inconsistent technique

   ii. variation in cardiac rate or rhythm

   iii. presence of mitral insufficiency

   iv. recirculation of indicator

   v. sudden change in patient's hemodynamic status

     a. i, ii, iii, and v

     b. ii and iv

   c. i only

   d. all of the above

8. The advantages of the thermodilution cardiac output method are:

   i. need for only one invasive catheter

   ii. rapid and reproducible serial determinations are possible

   iii. results are not affected by O_2 administration

   iv. accuracy in the presence of shunts and mitral valve disease

   v. absence of potential electrical hazard

      a. ii only

      b. i, ii, and iii

      c. i and iv

      d. all of the above

9. Cardiac index

   i. normalizes cardiac output by patient size

   ii. involves dividing cardiac output by BSA

   iii. of less than 2.2 liters/min/m² is associated with hypoperfusion

   iv. varies less between patients than does cardiac output

      a. i and ii

      b. iii only

      c. i, ii, iii, and iv

      d. none of the above

10. Refer back to the BSA nomogram (Fig. 2–6). A patient weighs 56.7 kg (125 lb) and is 170 cm (67 inches) tall. Her BSA is _____.

11. The patient above has a cardiac output of 4.9 liters/min. Her cardiac index is _____.

12. The same patient has a heart rate of 62 beats/min. Her stroke volume is _____.

Questions 13–17

A patient admitted to the ICU has the following hemodynamic parameters:

$$\begin{array}{ll} \underline{\text{HR:}} & \text{120 beats/min} \\ \underline{\text{RA:}} & \text{3 mmHg} \\ \text{PA:} & \text{19 mmHg} \end{array}$$

BP: 115/90 mmHg
PCWP: 5 mmHg
CO: 3.8 liters/min

13. His MAP is _____.

14. His SV is _____.

15. His SVR is _____.

16. His PVR is _____.

17. His LVSW is _____.

18. In measuring SVR, we are actually determining:
   a. pulmonary resistance
   b. preload
   c. LVEDP
   d. afterload

19. An abnormally high SVR could be associated with:
   i. hypovolemia
   ii. cardiogenic shock
   iii. vasodilation
   iv. hyperthermia
      a. iii only
      b. ii only
      c. i, iii, and iv
      d. i and ii

20. Abnormally high PVR can occur due to:
   i. high wedge pressures
   ii. pulmonary hypertension
   iii. hypoxia
   iv. COPD
      a. i only
      b. ii and iii
      c. ii, iii, and iv
      d. all of the above

21. The average pressure generated by the *left* ventricle during a contraction is:
   a. mean pulmonary artery pressure minus CVP
   b. systolic arterial pressure minus PCWP

c. systolic arterial pressure minus CVP

d. cardiac output divided by heart rate

22. Stroke work is affected by:

    i. SVR

    ii. preload

    iii. afterload

    iv. heart rate

        a. i and iii

        b. ii, iii, and iv

        c. ii only

        d. all of the above

23. Ventricular function curves can be generated by plotting which of the following parameters against PCWP?

    i. CI

    ii. SVI

    iii. LVSWI

    iv. HR

        a. iii only

        b. i only

        c. i, ii, iii

        d. all of the above

24. The ventricular function curve can be shifted upwards (augmented) directly by:

    a. increased contractility

    b. decreased contractility

    c. increased PCWP

    d. decreased PCWP

25. The ventricular function curve can be shifted downwards (depressed) by:

    a. increased contractility

    b. decreased contractility

    c. increased PCWP

    d. decreased PCWP

Section 2 Quiz Answers

The bracketed numbers following each answer indicate the pages where discussions for each question can be found.

1. c [42]
2. c [43]
3. a [40]
4. b [45]
5. d [46]
6. $\dfrac{5.3 + 5.5 + 5.6}{3}$ = 5.47 liters/min [51]
7. a [47]
8. b [47]
9. c [52]
10. 1.65 m^2 [52]
11. 4.9 liters/min ÷ 1.65 m^2 = 2.97 liters/min/m^2 [52]
12. 4.9 liters/min ÷ 62 beats/min = 79 ml [53]
13. $\dfrac{(115 \text{ mmHg} + 2(90 \text{ mmHg})}{3}$ = 98.3 mmHg [20]
14. 3.8 liters/min ÷ 120 beats/min = 31.7 ml [53]
15. $\dfrac{(98.3 \text{ mmHg} - 3 \text{ mmHg}) \times 80}{3.8 \text{ liters/min}}$ = 2006 dynes/sec/cm^5 [54]
16. $\dfrac{(19 \text{ mmHg} - 5 \text{ mmHg}) \times 80}{3.8 \text{ liters/min}}$ = 295 dynes/sec/cm^5 [56]
17. (115 mmHg − 5 mmHg) × 79 ml × 0.0136 = 47.4 g-m/beat [57]
18. d [54]
19. d [55]
20. c [56]
21. b [57]
22. d [56]
23. c [58]

24. a [59]
25. b [59]

If you had any incorrect answers, go back and review the areas you had difficulty with. Then come back and try those questions again. Once you feel that you fully understand the material covered in this section, proceed to Section 3.

Section 2 References

1. Altman PL, Dittmers DS (eds): Respiration and Circulation. Biological Handbooks. Bethesda, Md: Federation of American Societies for Experimental Biology, 1971
2. American Edwards Laboratories: Understanding hemodynamic measurements made with the Swan-Ganz catheter. Santa Ana, Calif: American Edwards Laboratories, 1979
3. Baele PL, McMichan JC, Marsh HM, et al: Continuous monitoring of mixed venous oxygen saturation in critically ill patients. Anesth Analg, 61:513, 1982
4. Forrester JS, Diamond G, Chatterjee K, Swan HJC: Medical therapy of myocardial infarction by application of hemodynamic subsets. N Engl J Med 295:, 1976
5. Ganz W, Donoso, R, Marcus HS: A new technique for measurement of cardiac output by thermodilution in man. Am J Cardiol 27:392, 1971
6. Jansen JRC, Schreuder JJ, Bogaard JM, et al: Thermodilution technique for measurement of cardiac output during artificial ventilation. J Appl Physiol 50:584, 1981
7. Levett JM, Replogle RL: Thermodilution cardiac output: A critical analysis and review of the literature. J Surg Res 27:392, 1978
8. Mueller H, Ayres S, Giannelli S, et al: Trans NY Sci Ser II, 34(4):309, 1972
9. Nelson LD, Houtchens BA: Automatic vs. manual injections for thermodilution cardiac output determinations. Crit Care Med 10:190, 1982
10. Nishikawa T, Dohi S: Slowing of heart rate during cardiac output measurement by thermodilution. Anaesthesiology 57:583, 1982
11. Shapiro HM, Smith G, Pribble AH, et al: Errors in sampling pulmonary arterial blood with a Swan–Ganz catheter. Anaesthesiology 40:291, 1974
12. Snyder JV, Powner DJ: Effects of mechanical ventilation on the measurement of cardiac output by thermodilution. Crit Care Med 10:677, 1982
13. Swan HJC, Ganz W: Hemodynamic measurement in clinical practice: A decade in review. J Am Coll Cardiol 1:103, 1983
14. Todd MM: Atrial fibrillation induced by the right atrial injection of cold fluids during thermodilution cardiac output determination: A case report. Anaesthesiology 59:253, 1983

15. Wong M, Skulsy A, Moon E: Loss of indicator in the thermodilution technique. Cathet Cardiovasc Diagn 4:103, 1978
16. Yang SS, Bentivaglio LG, Maranhan V, et al: From Cardiac Catheterization Data to Hemodynamic Parameters, 2nd ed. Philadelphia: F. A. Davis, 1978

Clinical Applications of Hemodynamic Measurements

In this section your previous experience with and knowledge of hemodynamic monitoring, along with the information provided by Sections 1 and 2, are brought together. We shall now look at how these hemodynamic measurements can be helpful in the clinical setting.

The purpose of this section is not to teach you everything about each specific clinical condition. Rather, it is to focus on the hemodynamic changes that occur with these conditions and explain what you will see in terms of hemodynamic parameters and how the use of these hemodynamic parameters can guide therapeutic intervention.

INDICATIONS FOR HEMODYNAMIC MONITORING

We have been concentrating on hemodynamic measurements made invasively, specifically through the use of a balloon-tipped flow-directed pulmonary artery catheter. It is important to remember that the monitoring of hemodynamic status does not begin and end with the pulmonary artery catheter. The purpose of hemodynamic monitoring is to assess the adequacy of circulation in the patient. By assessing your patient's level of consciousness, skin color and temperature, blood pressure, urine output, and heart rate you are assessing his or her hemodynamic performance. These are valuable assessments and should be carried out on all patients. These parameters are, however, slow indicators of change in hemodynamic status, requiring the passage of time before changes are apparent. There are many instances when the use of pulmonary artery pressure monitoring is indicated to provide rapid, beat-by-beat information on the patient's hemodynamic status, and to allow for rapid

77

response to changes with appropriate therapeutic interventions. Indications for the use of the pulmonary artery catheter include[2]:

- Acute heart failure
- Differentiation of ruptured ventricular septum from mitral regurgitation
- Cardiac tamponade
- Severe hypovolemia
- Complex circulatory situations, e.g., burn patients
- Adult respiratory distress syndrome
- Gram-negative sepsis
- Drug intoxication
- Acute renal failure
- Hemorrhagic pancreatitis
- Management of high-risk surgical patients
  - History of pulmonary or cardiac disease
  - Fluid shifts (extensive abdominal surgery)
- Management of high-risk obstetric patients
  - History of cardiac disease
  - Severe pregnancy-induced hypertension
  - Abruptio placentae

Although there are no absolute contraindications to the use of pulmonary artery catheters, it is important to weigh the benefit of use against the possible complications, especially in the case of patients with recurrent septicemia or hypercoagulable states. Table 3–1 lists the potential complications of hemodynamic monitoring. When a pulmonary artery catheter is being inserted into a patient with a complete left bundle branch block, special attention to ECG monitoring is necessary, as the risk of complete heart block is somewhat increased.[2] Special care in ECG monitoring of patients with a history of tachyarrhythmias (e.g., Wolff–Parkinson–White syndrome) or ventricular arrhythmias is necessary, as the insertion

TABLE 3–1. POTENTIAL COMPLICATIONS OF HEMODYNAMIC MONITORING WITH PULMONARY ARTERY CATHETERS

Related to Insertion	Related to Catheter Itself
Multiple insertion attempts	Atrial or ventricular dysrhythmias
Hematoma at insertion site	Perforation of atrial or ventricular wall
Arterial puncture	Pulmonary embolus (catheter, air, blood clot)
Local infection	Sepsis
Pneumothorax	Pulmonary artery injury
Hemothorax	Pulmonary infarction
Valvular damage	

procedure can cause recurrence of these arrhythmias. It is always necessary to have emergency resuscitation equipment on hand when a pulmonary artery catheter is being inserted.

PEDIATRIC HEMODYNAMIC MONITORING

The principles of hemodynamic monitoring that have been reviewed also apply to pediatric patients. The indications for invasive hemodynamic monitoring in children may differ, however, as children tend to have different medical problems from those of adults. For example, primary pump failure is unusual in children but heart failure may follow cardiac surgery, myocarditis, obstructive left-sided cardiac lesions such as coarctation of the aorta and hypoplastic left heart syndrome, or large left-to-right intracardiac shunts.

Perhaps the most common indication for hemodynamic monitoring in children is after cardiac surgery. The types of surgical procedures carried out in children usually involve correction of congenital abnormalities and so are different from the surgical procedures usually performed on adults. The nature of the abnormality and the type of surgical procedure performed may influence the expected values for the monitored hemodynamic parameters.

Another difference between adult and pediatric hemodynamic monitoring concerns the size of the catheters and lines used. The small size of pediatric lines makes them especially prone to occlusion. The size of the patient is also an important factor because hemodynamic parameters such as left ventricular end-diastolic pressure (LVEDP) will change more rapidly for a given change in intravascular volume in a small child than in an adult. There are many other differences between hemodynamic monitoring in adults and children but they are too numerous to be covered in detail here. The interested reader is encouraged to consult a textbook of pediatric cardiology for further information.

HEMODYNAMIC PARAMETERS SEEN
WITH SPECIFIC CLINICAL CONDITIONS

Myocardial Infarction
Hemodynamic monitoring can provide valuable information about ventricular performance in the patient with acute myocardial infarction (MI). Not only can this information guide us in optimizing ventricular function, it can also be used to assess myocardial oxygen demands. Maintenance of optimum ventricular function must be

balanced against the risk of increasing myocardial oxygen demands past the point where they can be met by the compromised coronary blood flow of the recently infarcted myocardium. If myocardial oxygen demand increases past this point, further myocardial damage can occur, resulting in further depression of ventricular function.

The major determinants of myocardial oxygen demands are afterload, heart rate, and myocardial contractility. The hemodynamic parameters that assess these functions are:

1. Afterload—systemic vascular resistance (SVR), systolic blood pressure (BP)
2. Heart rate (HR)
3. Contractility—left ventricular stroke volume index (LVSWI) and pulmonary capillary wedge pressure (PCWP) plotted as ventricular function curves

An increase in any of these hemodynamic parameters signifies an increase in myocardial oxygen demand. Therefore, any effort to improve the patient's cardiac function must be weighed against the possibility of increasing myocardial oxygen demands and inducing further cardiac ischemia.

Since patients with an acute MI vary greatly in terms of ventricular function, a list of hemodynamic parameter values expected with an MI cannot be predicted. However, patients can be classified into one of five groups, depending on their ventricular function curve (Fig. 3–1).[28] This classification can be utilized in the development of therapeutic and prognostic guidelines for each patient.

Some patients may demonstrate a normal ventricular function curve: normal stroke work and PCWP. Prognosis is very good and obviously no hemodynamic therapy is required.

Patients in group 1 have slightly abnormal ventricular performance: stroke work slightly low and PCWP slightly elevated. Again, prognosis is good and usually no hemodynamic therapy is required.

Patients in group 2 demonstrate moderate derangement of ventricular function: stroke work is low and PCWP is elevated. Therapeutic intervention in these cases would be aimed at maintaining PCWP at the level at which stroke work is optimized but pulmonary congestion is avoided.

Patients in group 3 are in cardiogenic shock: stroke work and cardiac output are low, resulting in tissue hypoperfusion. PCWP is markedly elevated, resulting in pulmonary edema in many cases. Again, therapeutic intervention is aimed at maintaining PCWP at the level that optimizes stroke work, shifting the ventricular function curve upwards by increasing contractility and increasing cardiac output by decreasing systemic vascular resistance (afterload). Prognosis is poor, and early treatment is necessary to maintain

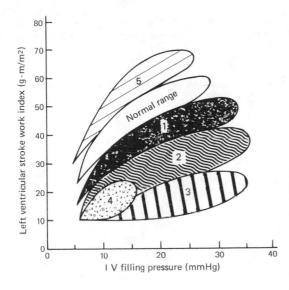

Figure 3–1. Classification of patients with acute myocardial infarction according to their position on the ventricular function curve. *(From Walinsky P: Acute hemodynamic monitoring. Heart Lung 6:840, 1977, with permission.)*

optimum tissue perfusion. (Refer to page 85 for more discussion on cardiogenic shock.)

Patients in group 4 may be clinically indistinguishable from group 3 patients. The difference lies in the fact that these patients are hypovolemic: stroke work and cardiac output are low (resulting in tissue hypoperfusion) and PCWP is low. This hypovolemic state may be due to use of diuretic agents, nausea and vomiting, or generalized dehydration. Therapeutic intervention includes careful volume expansion. Special care must be taken when volume-replenishing these patients as they usually have stiff, noncompliant ventricles and PCWP may increase rapidly with only moderate increases in circulating volume. For this reason, volume loading should be carried out slowly, with close monitoring of ventricular function. With resolution of the hypovolemic state, these patients may demonstrate group 3 ventricular function curves and therapeutic interventions should be carried out accordingly.

Patients in group 5 have hyperdynamic ventricular function: stroke work is elevated and PCWP is normal. The hyperdynamic state can be caused by hypertension, anxiety, or pain. This results in increased myocardial oxygen demand and may result in increased myocardial ischemia. Therapeutic intervention is aimed at reducing the causative hypertension, anxiety, or pain and, by so doing, decreasing myocardial oxygen demands.

Shock States

Shock is defined as "a syndrome produced by capillary hypoperfusion, resulting in the delivery to the cells of oxygen and nutrients in quantities inadequate for the maintenance of normal cell function."[3] Shock can be categorized according to the primary defect that produced it, that is, hypovolemic, cardiogenic, and vasogenic shock.[23]

Hypovolemic Shock. Hypovolemic shock is any shock that results from excessive loss of intravascular fluid volume. This type of shock can be divided into two categories:

1. Hemorrhagic shock
2. Nonhemorrhagic hypovolemic shock

Hemorrhagic shock is one of the most common forms of clinical shock. It implies a decrease in intravascular fluid volume related to loss of whole blood.

Nonhemorrhagic hypovolemic shock refers to a decrease in intravascular fluid volume secondary to losses from the interstitial space (e.g., pancreatitis, intraabdominal, third-space fluid loss, prolonged vomiting, and diarrhea). Since losses from the interstitial space are often occult (not visually apparent), it is easy to forget the potential for shock related to these losses. It is important to remember that prolonged or sustained loss of any body fluid will lead to hypovolemia and the potential for shock.

Hemodynamic parameters seen in hypovolemic shock reflect not only the decrease in circulating intravascular volume but also the body's attempt to compensate for this decrease. These compensatory mechanisms are largely related to the increase in sympathetic outflow that occurs when arterial baroreceptors detect a decrease in blood pressure (refer back to page 25).

Compensation includes arteriolar constriction in an attempt to maintain an adequate mean arterial pressure (MAP). Vasoconstriction occurs mainly in the skin and renal and splanchnic vessels, with little or no constriction of cerebral and cardiac vessels. In this way blood flow is directed preferentially to the brain and heart. Decreased venous capacitance results in an increase in venous return to the heart in an attempt to increase preload. Preload is also supported by the shift of blood from the splanchnic to systemic circulation that results from the generalized vasoconstriction. Tachycardia and increased contractility occur in an effort to maintain the cardiac output.

Decreased blood flow to the kidney results in minimal urine production due to decreased glomerular filtration rate and renal plasma flow. This, along with increased antidiuretic hormone (ADH) and aldosterone production induced by impaired renal blood flow (refer back to page 26), increases intravascular volume by the conservation of both sodium and water. Low capillary hydrostatic pressure and increased plasma protein production result in the shifting of fluid from extravascular spaces into the capillaries.

The primary problem in hypovolemic shock is a decrease in intravascular volume; this being the case, one would expect that mean right atrial ($\overline{RA}$) pressure and PCWP would be low in these patients. The generalized vasoconstriction along with the other compensatory mechanisms, however, may result in a normal or even elevated $\overline{RA}$ and PCWP, indicating that although total volume has decreased, the increase in vascular tone has compensated for this. When fluid loss exceeds the capacity for compensation by vasoconstriction, the $\overline{RA}$ pressure and PCWP will rapidly fall. Compensatory arteriolar constriction indicates that SVR is high. This is very important because the high SVR may result in "normal" arterial blood pressure despite the hypovolemia. This is an example of how blood pressure is not a good indicator of overall hemodynamic status. Although in early hypovolemic shock arterial blood pressure may be maintained by the high SVR, when $\overline{RA}$ pressure and PCWP fall so does cardiac output; eventually SVR will no longer be able to compensate and arterial blood pressure will fall. Pulmonary vascular resistance usually remains normal, except in the presence of other factors, such as hypoxia, pulmonary embolism, or chronic pulmonary disease, in which case PVR may be elevated.

The ventricular function curves of these patients can shift upwards, downwards, or may remain normal. Upward shift would be caused by release of catecholamines that increase myocardial contractility as well as increasing heart rate and enhancing vasoconstriction. The increased SVR (afterload) can further decrease cardiac output. The low-volume state (low PCWP) places the patient low on the curve. Mixed venous oxygen content will be reduced and the arterial–venous difference in oxygen content (a-v DO_2) will be increased due to the decreased cardiac output and inadequate tissue perfusion.

Treatment of hypovolemic shock is directed towards replacing intravascular volume and correcting the problem that led to hypovolemia. If the patient has a very low blood pressure, vasopressor agents may be used as a short-term therapy to maintain perfusion of vital organs by further increasing SVR. This results in a further decrease in tissue perfusion, however, so fluid resuscitation must be carried out concurrently and vasopressors used for the shortest possible length of time.

Controversy continues as to the best type of solution for fluid resuscitation in cases of hypovolemic shock, that is, colloid versus noncolloid fluids. Whatever the solution used, administration should be guided by $\overline{RA}$ pressure and PCWP. Fluid should be given until the $\overline{RA}$ pressure and/or PCWP reach the maximum level possible without inducing pulmonary congestion or cardiac decompensation. MAP may increase before $\overline{RA}$ pressure or PCWP increases significantly but hypovolemia is probably still present until $\overline{RA}$

pressure and $\overline{\text{PA}}$ PCWP reach normal levels. When fluid replacement is adequate, $\overline{\text{RA}}$ pressure and PCWP may start to rise quickly and further fluid administration should be titrated to maintain the patient at his or her optimum level.

Vasogenic Shock. The mechanism behind vasogenic shock is severe vasodilation resulting in a *relative* state of hypovolemia because the normal blood volume is inadequate in terms of filling the expanded vascular compartment. This vasodilation may be induced by several mechanisms. In anaphylactic shock histamine is released in response to an antigen–antibody reaction. Histamine causes vasodilation and increased capillary permeability, resulting in hypovolemia. Deep anesthesia may depress the vasomotor centers of the brain, resulting in loss of neural control of the vasculature and generalized vasodilation.

The most common clinical form of vasogenic shock is septic shock. Septic shock is characterized by the presence of pathogenic microorganisms and/or their toxins in the blood, resulting in hypotension and decreased tissue perfusion. Patients in critical-care settings have an increased likelihood of developing serious infections that can progress to septic shock. The use of invasive lines, endotracheal intubation and ventilation, and also the fact that many critically ill patients are unable to mount a normal defense against infection, make septic shock a potential hazard for these patients.

The pathophysiology of septic shock is not entirely clear. Almost any microorganism can cause sepsis but septic shock is most often associated with gram-negative organisms.[29] Gram-negative bacilli have cell walls that contain a complex lipopolysaccharide that has been identified as an endotoxin. When endotoxins are released into the circulation, the endothelium of blood vessels becomes damaged. This damage activates a complex pathway, which results in liberation of *kinins*. Kinins are polypeptides that produce vasodilation and increased permeability of capillaries.[24] Platelet breakdown also occurs and results in the release of *serotonin* and *histamine* into the circulation, which causes added vasodilation and increased capillary permeability, accentuating the action of the kinins.[20]

In the early stages of septic shock the patient presents with a hyperdynamic picture. The patient appears warm and flushed; this stage of septic shock is often called the "warm phase." The SVR is low because of the generalized vasodilation. Cardiac output increases in the face of this decreased afterload, and the ventricular function curve is shifted upwards. RA pressure and PCWP are abnormally low because of the relative hypovolemia induced by vasodilation. The a-v DO_2 is decreased more than would be expected, even with the increase in cardiac output. This occurs because of shunting of blood past capillary beds. This shunting means that even though the blood may be carrying adequate amounts of oxygen and nutrients, the tissues are not receiving these nutrients and a state of tissue hypoperfusion exists. Blood pressure at this stage is supported by the increased cardiac output and may be normal or slightly low.

At this stage in septic shock, fluid administration is required to "fill up" the enlarged vascular compartment. Fluid administration can be guided by $\overline{RA}$ pressure and PCWP. The goal of treatment is to reach and maintain a PCWP that will optimize cardiac output. A cardiac output within "normal" range is not adequate in these patients. Their increased vascular capacity requires a higher than normal cardiac output in order to maximize tissue perfusion. Of course it is essential to identify and treat the cause of the sepsis as soon as possible.

If septic shock persists, the patient will progress from the "warm phase" into the later "cold phase." The cold phase is characterized by the patient becoming pale, cold, and clammy. Effective circulatory volume falls even further due to continued vasodilation and fluid shift from the vascular to the interstitial and intracellular compartments. In this phase, the ineffective vascular volume leads to increased sympathetic outflow and peripheral vasoconstriction. Cardiac failure occurs related to increased myocardial oxygen demands. Myocardial oxygen demands increase due to increased heart rate, increased afterload, and the presence of high levels of catecholamines in response to sympathetic stimulation. Coronary artery perfusion pressure is low due to inadequate cardiac output.

PCWP falls and cardiac output starts to decrease but the low a-v DO_2 persists. Cardiac output is further reduced due to the increased afterload, and depressed myocardial contractility shifts the ventricular function curve downwards. As with hypovolemic shock, the patient will be on the low end of the curve (low PCWP). Treatment at this stage involves fluid administration to increase PCWP and attempts to improve cardiac output and shift the ventricular function curve upwards by decreasing afterload and increasing myocardial contractility. As always, the underlying problem must be dealt with, including identification and appropriate treatment of the causative microorganism.

Cardiogenic Shock. Decreased myocardial contractility is the mechanism behind cardiogenic shock. Myocardial contractility may be impaired due to loss of function of a critical amount of myocardium such as might occur with acute MI or severe cardiomyopathy, or due to mechanical factors that decrease left ventricular filling or systolic ejection of blood such as constrictive pericarditis, cardiac tamponade, mitral stenosis, or aortic stenosis. Acute myocardial infarction is the most common cause of cardiogenic shock, which usually results if at least 40% of the left ventricular myocardium has been impaired.[1] Further discussion of cardiogenic shock is restricted to shock due to acute MI.

Reduced left ventricular contractility results in decreased cardiac output due to decreased stroke volume. Since less blood is ejected per beat, more blood remains in the ventricle, thus increasing preload (PCWP). Up to a point, this increased PCWP (causing increased myocardial fiber stretch) can increase stroke volume and force of contraction (as per Starling's law of the heart). When the PCWP exceeds the optimum level, force of contraction and stroke work begin to fall. In response to the decreased cardiac output, SVR increases in an effort to maintain adequate mean arterial pressures. In other words, the body attempts to compensate for low cardiac output in the same manner as occurs with hypovolemic shock (see page 82). This increased SVR (afterload) also increases the work the heart must perform in order to pump blood, further taxing the already compromised ventricle and increasing myocardial oxygen demands. Despite the increased SVR and because of the impaired contractility of the ventricle, arterial blood pressure drops. The low cardiac output results in increased a-v DO_2 because blood remains in the capillaries for a relatively long period, allowing enhanced oxygen extraction. Pulmonary vascular resistance is normal or may be high in the presence of hypoxemia. The decreased contractility shifts the ventricular function curve downwards. The patient will be on the high end of the curve due to the high PCWP.

Therapeutic intervention is aimed at maintaining PCWP at the level of optimum stroke work and shifting the ventricular function curve upwards. Increasing contractility will accomplish this upward shift. Keep in mind, however, that increasing the contractility of the ventricle when it still has to pump against a very high afterload (SVR) can further tax the already compromised myocardium. Also, positive inotropic agents such as dopamine enhance the contractility of only *unimpaired* myocardium; therefore the larger the infarct, the smaller the effect. Afterload reduction is therefore a very important intervention in cardiogenic shock, as it decreases the resistance the heart must pump against and increases stroke volume. Reduction of afterload (decreasing SVR) also reduces PCWP, as a more dilated vasculature can accommodate more blood, thus decreasing venous return and preload.

Maintenance of optimum PCWP can be accomplished by the use of fluid administration and diuretic agents. The optimum range for PCWP varies from patient to patient but is usually between 15 and 18 mmHg.[13] If the patient's PCWP is greater than 18 mmHg and/or pulmonary congestion is present, the use of diuretic agents such as furosemide may be indicated. Furosemide reduces PCWP by increasing venous capacitance and by enhancing excretion of sodium and water by the kidneys. If, however, the patient's PCWP is less than 15 mmHg and he or she remains hypoperfused, careful administration of fluid may be required to raise the PCWP to a more optimal level. This may be necessary if the patient is started on an afterload-reducing agent such as nitroprusside. The decrease in afterload that occurs may decrease the PCWP below optimum, necessitating judicious fluid replacement.

Isolated PCWP determinations are not as helpful, in terms of guiding therapy as are serial measurements of PCWP and cardiac output, with calculation of hemodynamic indices such as SVR and LVSW. Only by continued monitoring of these parameters and by plotting ventricular function curves can optimum PCWP be determined and response to therapy evaluated.

Circulatory assist devices such as the intraaortic balloon pump (IABP) may be utilized in the setting of cardiogenic shock to improve ventricular function and to augment coronary and systemic arterial perfusion. IABP utilizes the principle of counterpulsation to provide diastolic augmentation and systolic unloading (afterload reduction). A balloon-equipped catheter is inserted into the femoral artery and advanced until it sits in the thoracic aorta below the origin of the left subclavian artery. The balloon is mechanically inflated during diastole and deflated just prior to the onset of ventricular systole (Fig. 3–2). An ECG sensing device and aortic waveform monitor are used to time inflation so that it occurs just after

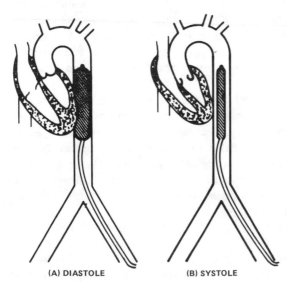

(A) DIASTOLE   (B) SYSTOLE

Figure 3–2. An intraaortic balloon pump in place within the thoracic aorta. The balloon is inflated during diastole (**A**) and deflated just prior to systole (**B**).

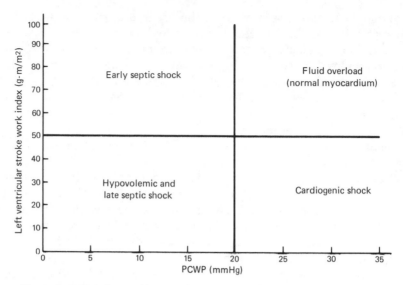

Figure 3–3. Relative positions on the ventricular function curve of patients in different types of shock.

the T wave on the ECG and coincides with the dicrotic notch (aortic valve closure) on the aortic waveform. Deflation coincides with the QRS complex on the ECG and the end-diastolic point on the aortic waveform.

Diastolic augmentation is provided by the actual inflation of the balloon (after closure of the aortic valve). This inflation acts as a pump that forces blood in a retrograde direction up the aortic arch and increases diastolic aortic pressure. In this way perfusion of the coronary arteries is augmented (since the coronary arteries receive most of their blood flow during diastole) and myocardial oxygen supply is improved. Mean arterial pressure also rises due to the increased antegrade diastolic pressure, thus generally improving systemic perfusion.

Systolic unloading (afterload reduction) is also achieved through the use of IABP. When the balloon deflates with the onset of ventricular systole, blood flows passively from the aortic arch into the thoracic aorta to fill the space formerly occupied by the inflated balloon. This lowers the blood volume in the aorta and reduces resistance to left ventricular ejection. Since afterload is reduced, the left ventricle can pump more effectively and myocardial oxygen demands are reduced.

IABP can be a valuable temporary method to assist the patient's circulation mechanically. It is an invasive measure, however, and has many potential complications, such as damage to the aorta, systemic embolization, balloon rupture, and the introduction of infection directly into the vascular system. It requires precise timing and skilled, knowledgeable personnel to achieve optimum results and prevent complications.

Figure 3–3 shows the relative positions of patients in different types of shock on the ventricular function curve.

Mitral Valve Disease

Normally PCWP reflects the pressure of the left atrium, which is the same as the pressures in the left ventricle during diastole (when the mitral valve is open). Under normal conditions the mitral valve closes during ventricular systole; therefore, ventricular systolic pressures do not affect the PCWP. As with the pressure waveform of the right atrium, the PCWP exhibits small positive deflections— the a wave representing atrial contraction and the v wave representing filling of the left atrium during isovolumic ventricular contraction (see Fig. 1–8). If the mitral valve is diseased and not closing properly, blood is pushed back up into the left atrium during ventricular systole. Instead of a small v wave, representing isovolumic ventricular contraction, a large v wave, representing backflow or regurgitation of blood into the left atrium during ventricular contraction, will be seen (Fig. 3–4). This will result in a high PCWP that is not representative of true LVEDP. To get a better indication of LVEDP the *diastolic* rather than mean value for PCWP can be obtained (Fig. 3–3). It is best to remember, however, that LVEDP estimation by PCWP is inaccurate in the presence of mitral valve disease.

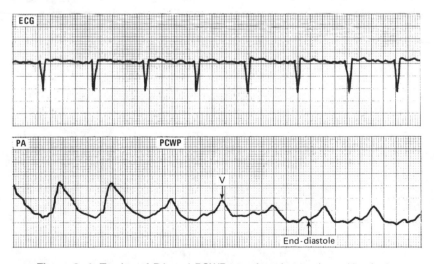

Figure 3–4. Tracing of PA and PCWP waveform in a patient with mitral regurgitation. Note prominent "v" wave. End-diastolic point is indicated.

If tissue perfusion is compromised in the patient with mitral valve disease, treatment is aimed at improving cardiac output. Afterload reduction, possibly by using sodium nitroprusside, will decrease the amount of resistance to blood flow into the systemic circulation and may consequently reduce the amount of regurgitant flow into the left atrium. As impedance to aortic flow diminishes, a larger fraction of the total left ventricular output will be ejected through the aorta and cardiac output will increase.

Ventricular Septal Defects

In the presence of a ventricular septal defect (VSD) blood is usually being shunted from the high-pressure left ventricle to the lower-pressure right ventricle during ventricular systole. Cardiac output may be reduced because part of the blood pumped by the left ventricle is going into the right ventricle rather than into the aorta. Since the right ventricle is receiving extra blood during systole, its preload is increased, as seen by increased RV diastolic and $\overline{RA}$ pressures.

More diagnostic of VSD, however, is a "step-up" in oxygen saturation from right atrium to pulmonary artery. Normally, the oxygen saturation of blood in the right atrium and pulmonary artery is the same. In VSD, however, oxygenated blood from the left ventricle is shunted into the right ventricle, and the oxygen saturation of the blood in the pulmonary artery is increased.

To detect this step-up pattern, simultaneous blood samples must be obtained from the right atrium (proximal port of PA catheter) and from the pulmonary artery (distal port). These samples are sent for blood-gas analysis and the results compared.

EXAMPLE:

A patient has RA and PA blood drawn for blood-gas analysis. The results show:

$$RA \ O_2 \ \text{saturation } 75\%$$
$$PA \ O_2 \ \text{saturation } 85\%$$

Since the blood has become more saturated with oxygen between the right atrium and the pulmonary artery, a ventricular septal defect is suspected.

Treatment includes the use of afterload-reducing agents to stabilize the patient by increasing forward blood flow and optimizing cardiac output.

Constrictive Pericarditis/Pericardial Tamponade

In constrictive pericarditis and pericardial tamponade there is increased pressure surrounding the heart that results in compromise of myocardial function. After the ventricles contract, the surrounding pericardial sac inhibits complete reexpansion of the ventricles. Ventricular filling is impaired and stroke volume decreases, reducing cardiac output. Since ventricular function is impaired and stroke volume is decreased, more blood remains in the ventricle after systole. Preload and therefore PCWP (left ventricle) and $\overline{RA}$ pressure (right ventricle) increase. Because the right ventricle is not as strong as the left ventricle, right ventricular filling is the first to be impaired and $\overline{RA}$ pressure will rise before PCWP. Signs of right ventricular failure such as increased jugular venous pressure and peripheral edema may be apparent. Eventually $\overline{RA}$ pressure and PCWP equalize. In severe tamponade, the ventricles can only contract slightly and all intracardiac pressures eventually equalize, dramatically compromising circulation. An increase in mean right atrial pressure and simultaneous decrease in mean arterial pressure during inspiration (during which venous return to the right atrium is increased and left atrial filling decreased) is characteristic of cardiac tamponade.

Treatment of these disorders consists of reducing the constriction around the heart. In chronic constrictive pericarditis surgical removal of the pericardium may be necessary if the patient is significantly compromised. Pericardiocentesis with removal of fluid from the pericardial sac is the treatment for cardiac tamponade.

Pulmonary Embolus

With the occurrence of significant pulmonary embolism, an acute increase in pulmonary vascular resistance (PVR) occurs as a result of obstruction to pulmonary blood flow and the release of local vasoconstricting factors by the lung. Consequently, PA systolic, diastolic, and mean pressures rise. Right ventricular failure may occur as a result of the high pressures within the pulmonary arteries (high right ventricular afterload) and may be associated with high RA pressures. Since the function of the left ventricle is not affected, PCWP will usually remain normal. In massive pulmonary embolism or in the presence of multiple smaller emboli, blood flow from pulmonary arteries to the left atrium may be impaired to a degree that results in decreased left ventricular filling, and therefore PCWP may actually be decreased. With the high PA diastolic pressure and normal PCWP, a right–left pressure gradient greater than 6 mmHg will be seen.

Hemodynamic monitoring can be helpful in distinguishing pulmonary embolism from acute myocardial infarction. Both of these disease entities may present with similar signs and symptoms, for example, chest pain and shortness of breath. However, myocardial infarction is usually associated with normal PVR and high PCWP and is not usually associated with right ventricular failure unless left ventricular failure is also present. The presence of elevated PVR and normal PCWP would suggest that pulmonary embolism has occurred.

Treatment of pulmonary embolism is based on supportive management of resulting pain, hypoxia, and right heart failure and removal of the embolus obstruction. Thrombolytic therapy, the use of agents such as streptokinase to break up the clots and remove the obstruction, may be used in life-threatening situations.

Mechanical Ventilation/PEEP

During spontaneous respiration intrapleural pressures become increasingly negative with inspiration. Mechanical ventilation reverses this normal physiologic effect because positive pressure inspiration creates increasingly positive intrapleural pressure. This increase in intrapleural pressure also increases intrathoracic pressure, which can alter the patient's hemodynamic status.[11]

Increased intrapleural pressure and increased resistance to blood flow due to compression of the heart and vena cava by high intrathoracic pressure result in decreased venous return to the heart. Decreased venous return results in decreased preload and reduced cardiac output.[12]

The addition of positive end-expiratory pressure (PEEP) accentuates the effects on hemodynamic status. The continuously increased intrathoracic pressure resulting from PEEP further reduces left ventricular filling and reduces preload. Preload may also be decreased as a result of increased impedance to blood flow through the lungs.[23] PEEP does not appear to reduce myocardial contractility.[16,17,21]

Although PEEP decreases cardiac output by reducing preload, measured PCWP may be elevated. This sounds like a contradiction since conventionally PCWP is used as an estimate of preload. To clarify this, we must remember that preload is defined as transmural pressure (see page 23), that is, the pressure within the ventricle (ventricular end diastolic pressure) minus the pressure outside the ventricle (pericardial pressure). If, by using PEEP, we dramatically increase the pressure outside of the ventricle more than we increase pressure within the ventricle, true preload will be decreased despite an increased ventricular end-diastolic pressure.

A hypothetical example may illustrate this concept: A patient is admitted to the Intensive Care Unit with respiratory failure and requires endotracheal intubation and mechanical ventilation. A pulmonary artery catheter is inserted and his PCWP is found to be 15 mmHg; we assume that his pericardial pressure is zero. PEEP is added and his PCWP is found to be 18 mmHg. If we imagine that the PEEP caused an increase in pericardial pressure of 5 mmHg, we can see that his true preload (LVEDP—pericardial pressure) is 18 − 5 = 13 mmHg and has actually decreased despite the increase in PCWP.

Pericardial pressure is difficult to measure at the bedside but recent research suggests that $\overline{RA}$ pressure correlates well with pericardial pressure.[25] Thus, PCWP minus $\overline{RA}$ pressure may provide a more reliable estimate of preload than what can be achieved by using PCWP alone.[26]

Adult Respiratory Distress Syndrome

In adult respiratory distress syndrome (ARDS), injury occurs at the microcirculatory level of the pulmonary capillary bed. Toxins are released that alter capillary and alveolar membranes. The pulmonary capillaries become "leaky"—more permeable to fluid and protein. Unlike in pulmonary edema of congestive heart failure, it is not increased hydrostatic pressures due to blood backup that cause the wet lungs of ARDS. Normal hydrostatic pressure will cause fluid leakage in ARDS due to the leaky pulmonary capillaries. Proteins also are able to leak out of the capillaries, resulting in decreased oncotic pressures within the capillaries and increased oncotic pressure in interstitial spaces. This causes further fluid leakage out of the capillaries, as the hydrostatic–oncotic pressure balance is upset. (Refer back to page 8 for review of intravascular pressure balance.) The result of this fluid and protein leakage is fluid extravasation into the lungs with decreased intravascular fluid volume. PCWP will be normal or low; this distinguishes ARDS from pulmonary edema due to congestive heart failure (where PCWP is high). The hypoxemia and decreased pulmonary compliance associated with ARDS may result in elevated PA systolic, diastolic, and mean pressures, as well as high PVR.

Treatment of ARDS consists of ventilatory support, which may include continuous PEEP as well as measures to ensure that optimum cardiac output is maintained. The use of corticosteroid hormones in ARDS remains controversial.

THE USE OF PHARMACOLOGIC AGENTS TO OPTIMIZE CARDIAC PERFORMANCE

The therapy of patients with hemodynamic abnormalities is aimed at optimizing cardiac performance so that adequate tissue perfusion and oxygenation is maintained while also maintaining the lowest possible myocardial oxygen demands. In some cases, for example, hypovolemic shock, this may be accomplished simply by the administration of adequate amounts of fluid to restore preload (LVEDP) to the optimum level. In other situations, as with cardiogenic shock, thereapy includes the administration of pharmacologic agents that alter preload, afterload, and contractility. Of course, treatment of arrhythmias, including brady- and tachyarrhythmias, is also essential in order to optimize cardiac function, but this will not be discussed here.

Agents that Affect Preload

Preload can be altered either by changing the amount of circulating volume or by changing the capacitance of the venous vasculature. The amount of circulating volume can be increased by the administration of fluids or can be decreased through the use of diuretic agents or phlebotomy. The capacitance of the blood vessels can be increased by the use of venodilating agents that will then decrease preload. Venous capacitance can be decreased through the use of agents that promote venoconstriction, but this is rarely done because fluid administration is a more effective means of increasing preload.

Diuretics. Diuretics are pharmacologic agents that increase the rate of urine formation. Although many diuretics do act directly on the kidney, direct action on the kidney is not necessary in order to produce a diuretic effect. Any drug that increases cardiac output may have a diuretic effect by increasing renal blood flow, which in turn enhances urine production.

One of the most potent diuretic agents is furosemide, a so-called loop diuretic that acts primarily by inhibiting chloride and sodium reabsorption in the ascending limb of the loop of Henle.[4,8] As well as decreasing intravascular volume, furosemide also causes venodilation, which further decreases preload and reduces pulmonary congestion.[7] The rapid onset of action seen with intravenous furosemide makes it a valuable therapeutic agent for the treatment of acute pulmonary edema and cardiogenic shock. The use of potent diuretic agents such as furosemide can, however, lead to excessive diuresis, which may result in hypovolemia and further compromise of the patient's hemodynamic status. Careful monitoring of PCWP and cardiac output as well as construction of ventricular function curves should be used to guide the administration of diuretic agents.

In addition to the potential for causing excessive diuresis leading to hypovolemia, potent diuretics such as furosemide may also cause serious electrolyte disturbances, such as hypokalemia, which may aggravate arrhythmias and cause further hemodynamic instability. Use of these drugs must be accompanied by careful assessment of the patient's electrolyte and fluid status and hemodynamic performance.

Venodilators. Organic nitrates such as nitroglycerin exert their vasodilating effects primarily on the venous vasculature, resulting in a decrease in preload.[18] Other vasodilators such as sodium nitroprusside produce dilation of both arterial and venous beds and result in reduction of afterload as well as preload. These drugs are reviewed in the following section, Agents that Affect Afterload.

Nitroglycerin, as well as reducing preload, also decreases pulmonary vascular resistance and reduces pulmonary congestion.[9] Myocardial oxygen demand is decreased through reduction of preload and oxygen supply may be enhanced by reduced pulmonary congestion, which facilitates improved gas exchange.

Nitroglycerin has a rapid onset of action and is a short-acting agent. Continuous drip intravenous nitroglycerine can be titrated to produce an optimum effect as assessed by serial PCWP and cardiac output determinations. Because rapid or excessive venodilation may cause unacceptable reductions in blood pressure, treatment must be monitored carefully and individualized in order to ensure appropriate reductions in preload.

Morphine is often used in cardiogenic shock and acute myocardial infarction to provide pain relief and sedation. It also appears to dilate pulmonary and systemic vascular beds, resulting in decreased preload. Dilation of resistance vessels also occurs to some degree, resulting in afterload reduction.

Agents that Affect Afterload

Patients in cardiogenic shock usually have elevated systemic vascular resistance due to compensatory sympathetic nervous system stimulation. In order to improve cardiac output it is often necessary to reduce afterload. Because high afterload also increases myocardial oxygen demand, afterload reduction is also important to decrease these demands and avoid further myocardial damage.

Nitroprusside is a directly acting intravenous drug that produces dilation of both venous and arterial beds,[18] resulting in decreased preload as well as decreased afterload. Although this generalized vasodilation can result in decreased systemic blood pressure, the concurrent increase in cardiac output may counterbalance this effect and blood pressure may not change significantly. If blood pressure does fall dramatically, it is often due to excessive reduction of preload, and judicious fluid administration may restore the PCWP to optimal levels. If the patient's PCWP is below optimal levels before nitroprusside therapy is started, fluids should be carefully administered to bring filling pressure to an optimum level prior to initiating afterload reduction.

Nitroprusside is an extremely potent vasodilator, with a rapid onset of action and a very short half-life. The patient's blood pressure can be "adjusted" to a specific level by carefully titrating the nitroprusside infusion rate. Serial determination of PCWP, cardiac output, and derived parameters, especially SVR, can be used to guide the administration of this drug. For these reasons nitroprusside has become a valuable therapeutic tool in the management of cardiogenic shock and in other conditions, such as mitral regurgitation, where high SVR impairs cardiac output. Sodium nitroprusside is only available in intravenous preparations and must be administered meticulously to avoid dramatic, undesirable reductions in blood pressure. Some patients, once stabilized, may require ongoing afterload reduction. An oral preparation such as prazosin may be used in this situation.

Afterload reduction can also be undertaken with α-adrenergic antagonist agents such as phentolamine. Phentolamine exerts its dilating effect primarily on the arterioles and it has less effect on preload than does nitroprusside. It also tends to cause tachycardia, which may be undesirable in the patient with a precarious oxygen supply–demand status.[5] The use of an intraaortic balloon pump can also effectively decrease afterload (see page 87).

Agents that Affect Contractility

In order to shift the ventricular function curve upwards, contractility must be increased. Although this may be associated with increased myocardial oxygen demand, the patient in cardiogenic shock may need more than afterload reduction and optimum preload in order to achieve an adequate cardiac output. In these cases, the cautious use of drugs that increase contractility (positive inotropic agents) may be indicated.

In order to minimize the increases in myocardial oxygen demand, it is important to use a positive inotropic agent that has a minimal effect on increasing heart rate and increasing systemic vascular resistance. Table 3–2 describes the relative hemodynamic actions of specific catecholamines.

Two of the most commonly used cathecholamines are dopamine and dobutamine. Dopamine is a naturally occurring catecholamine that acts on α- and β-adrenergic receptors as well as specific dopamine receptors.[15] The effects of dopamine are dose related.

At low doses, dopaminergic effects predominate, causing dilation of renal arteries and an increase in renal blood flow[14]; at higher doses dopamine stimulates β_1 receptors in the heart, causing increased myocardial contractility and improved cardiac output.

As dopamine dosage increases even further, stimulation of α receptors occurs, resulting in peripheral vasoconstriction and increased afterload. Blood pressure may increase because of the increased SVR but cardiac output may fall due to decreased stroke volume resulting from increased resistance to ventricular ejection.

TABLE 3–2. RELATIVE HEMODYNAMIC ACTIONS OF CATECHOLAMINES

Receptor	Response to Stimulation	Naturally Occurring			Synthetic		
		Norepinephrine	Epinephrine	Dopamine	Isoproterenol	Phenylephrine	Dobutamine
α	Vasoconstriction of cutaneous, skeletal muscle intestinal and renal vasculature	↑↑	low dose ± higher dose ↑↑	low dose ± increased effect as dosage increases	—	↑↑	±
β₁	Positive inotropic effect	↑→	↑↑	low doses ± higher doses ++	↑↑	↑↑	↑↑↑
	Positive chronotropic effect	↑	↑↑	↑↑	↑↑	±	
β₂	Bronchodilation vasodilation of mesenteric and skeletal muscle vasculature	—	low dose ↑↑ higher dose ↑	—	↑↑ ↑↑↑	—	±
Dopaminergic	Vasodilation of mesenteric and renal vasculature	—	—	low doses ↑↑	—	—	—

±, minimal effect; ↑, increase (small); ↓, decrease; —, no effect; ↑↓, may increase or decrease; ↑↑, increase (moderate); ↑↑↑, increase (marked)

Because the heart must pump against a higher resistance, myocardial oxygen demand increases. Tachyarrhythmias may also occur at high doses of dopamine, further increasing myocardial oxygen demand.

Dobutamine is a synthetic catecholamine that is also used as a positive inotropic agent in cardiogenic shock. Like dopamine, it is administered by continuous intravenous infusion and must be used with caution. Dobutamine exerts a potent positive inotropic effect on the myocardium but, unlike dopamine, is not associated with significant increases in SVR, even at high doses. Moreover, it does not tend to cause tachyarrhythmias. For these reasons dobutamine may result in less of an increase in myocardial oxygen demand than occurs with dopamine.[27]

The use of afterload-reducing agents in combination with positive inotropic drugs may provide optimum cardiac output. The simultaneous use of agents such as sodium nitroprusside and low to moderate doses of dopamine (or dobutamine) can enhance the reduction of preload and afterload as well as increase contractility. The equation

$$MAP = CO \times SVR$$

can be used to illustrate the advantages of using these agents concurrently. If afterload reduction alone results in an increase in cardiac output that is not sufficient to compensate for the decrease in SVR, MAP will fall. The positive inotropic effect of dopamine may improve cardiac output sufficiently to maintain the MAP while keeping afterload low. On the other hand, if dopamine is used alone, it stimulates the myocardium to contract more forcefully against a high SVR. High doses of dopamine may indeed make the SVR even higher. This results in increased myocardial oxygen demands in the presence of an already compromised myocardium. The addition of sodium nitroprusside decreases SVR and enhances the effect of dopamine by increasing stroke volume and thereby increasing cardiac output. Decreased afterload also results in decreased myocardial oxygen demand. The decrease in preload that occurs with nitroprusside therapy will further enhance cardiac output (providing that intravascular volume is adequate). In these ways, combination therapy can optimize cardiac function in cardiogenic shock.

Summary of Important Concepts in Section 3

The following is a table of *expected hemodynamic parameter values* in specific clinical conditions:

Clinical Condition	PCWP	RA	CO	SVR	PVR	a-v Do$_2$
Hypovolemic shock	↓	↓	↓	↑	—	↑
Septic shock (early)	↓	↓	↑	↓	—	↓
(late)	↓	↓	↓	↑	—	↓
Cardiogenic shock	↑	↑	↓	↑	—	↑
Pulmonary embolus	?↓	↑	↓	—	↑	—
Pericardial tamponade	↑	↑	↓	↑	—	—
ARDS	↓	↓	↓	↑	↑	—
Mechanical ventilation	?↑	—	↓	↑	↑	—
Mitral valve disease	↑	—	↓	↑	—	—
VSD	—	↑	↓	↑	—	—

KEY: ↑, increased; ↓, decreased; —, neither increased nor decreased specifically; ?, may be increased (or decreased) in some cases.

Patients with *myocardial infarction* vary greatly in terms of ventricular function. The use of *ventricular function curves* can be helpful in placing these patients into one of five prognostic categories.

Case Studies

Case 1

Mr. C. is a 66-year-old man who came to the Emergency Department by ambulance with severe retrosternal chest pain unrelieved by four nitroglycerin tablets. He has a history of previous myocardial infarction 2 years ago. A 12-lead ECG done in the Emergency Department showed S-T segment elevation in leads I, aVL, and V_3 to V_6, with q waves in leads II, III, and aVF. Blood was drawn for routine admission lab work and cardiac isoenzymes. An intravenous line was established and 5% dextrose in water solution was hung to keep the vein open. His pain was relieved with 7.5 mg of morphine sulfate given intravenously. Mr. C. was transferred to the Coronary Care Unit with the diagnosis of acute myocardial infarction. You are assigned to care for Mr. C.

1. Considering Mr. C.'s current diagnosis and past history, what complication of acute MI will you be particularly alert for?
2. Your ongoing assessment of Mr. C. includes assessment of the adequacy of his cardiac output. Since Mr. C. does not have invasive hemodynamic monitoring lines in place, how will you assess his cardiac output?

Your findings on initial assessment of Mr. C. include the following:

- *Vital signs:* BP 135/85 mmHg, HR 95 beats/min, respiration 16/min, temperature 37°C.
- *Central nervous system (CNS):* Alert and oriented. Moves all limbs well. Slightly anxious but responding well to reassurance and explanations.
- *Cardiovascular system (CVS):* Normal sinus rhythm with no extrasystoles. Heart sounds, S_1, S_2 with no extra sounds or murmurs heard. Extremities are slightly cool, but otherwise skin is warm and dry. No jugular venous distention (JVD) is noted. There is no peripheral or sacral edema. He remains free of chest pain.
- *Respiratory system:* Patient is on 3 liters/min O_2 per nasal prongs. No dyspnea or respiratory distress. No cyanosis. Chest is clear with adequate air entry throughout.

- *Gastrointestinal system (GI)*: Abdomen is soft and nontender. No masses on palpation. Bowel sounds are present.
- *Genitourinary system (GU)*: Has not voided since arrival in hospital (2 hours previously).

Four hours later you note that Mr. C.'s heart rate has climbed to 115 beats/min. His assessment remains unchanged and he denies further chest pain and does not appear to be more anxious than previously.

3. What might this increase in heart rate be indicative of?

Subsequently, Mr. C. develops crackles in his lung fields bilaterally, and he becomes cool and clammy. His BP is 100/80 mmHg, HR 120 beats/min, respirations 20/min. A pulmonary artery catheter is inserted, as is an arterial line and Foley catheter. Upon insertion of the PA catheter the following pressures are recorded:

$\overline{RA}$:	10 mmHg
PA systolic:	40 mmHg
PA diastolic:	26 mmHg
$\overline{PA}$:	31 mmHg
PCWP:	24 mmHg

4. Interpret these results.

Thermodilution cardiac output determination is carried out and his cardiac output is found to be 3.5 liters/min. His heart rate is 125 beats/min and his BP is 100/80 mmHg. (Mr. C. is 163 cm tall and weighs 70 kg.)

5. Calculate and interpret the following parameters for Mr. C.:

   Mean arterial pressure (MAP)
   Cardiac index (CI) (refer to Dubois BSA nomogram, Fig. 2–6)
   Stroke volume (SV)
   Systemic vascular resistance (SVR)
   Pulmonary vascular resistance (PVR)
   Left ventricular stroke work (LVSW)
   Right ventricular stroke work (RVSW)

6. What would be appropriate aims of treatment for Mr. C. and how might they be achieved?

Intravenous nitroprusside is initiated at 0.5 μg/kg/min and is increased to 2.5 μg/kg/min over the next 2 hours.

7. What properties of nitroprusside make careful, continuous blood pressure monitoring with an arterial line essential when using this agent?

Mr. C.'s mean arterial pressure remains relatively stable during his therapy with nitroprusside. His PCWP decreases to 19 mmHg and his CO increases to 4.1 liters/min.

8. Why did the MAP not fall dramatically when nitroprusside was given?

Case 1 Answer Key

1. Pump failure. Since Mr. C. has had previous myocardial damage, this acute MI may further reduce the pumping efficiency of his heart, leading to congestive heart failure and perhaps cardiogenic shock. Other possible complications include ventricular arrhythmias.

2. Your noninvasive assessment of Mr. C.'s cardiac output should include

   - Heart rate and rhythm and cardiac auscultation for the presence of extra heart sounds
   - Blood pressure
   - Skin color and temperature
   - Level of consciousness
   - Urine output
   - Ausculation of lungs for presence of crackles and other adventitious sounds
   - Assessment of jugular venous pressure/distention (JVD)
   - Assessment of limbs and sacrum for edema

3. The increase in heart rate may indicate that Mr. C.'s heart is pumping less effectively. In order to maintain cardiac output in the face of decreased stroke volume, his heart rate has increased.

4. All of these pressures are elevated above normal values. The R-L gradient is less than 6 ($26 - 24 = 2$), indicating that the elevated PA pressures have a cardiac, rather than pulmonary, cause. Mr. C.'s bibasilar crackles are a result of the high PCWP. These values are compatible with a patient in cardiac failure or a patient who has been fluid overloaded.

5. $\text{MAP} = [100 + 2(80)] \div 3 = 87$

   $\text{CI} = 3.5 \text{ liters/min} \div 1.75 \text{ m}^2 = 2.0 \text{ liters/min/m}^2$

   $\text{SV} = 3.5 \text{ liters/min} \div 125 \text{ beats/min} = 0.028 \text{ liters or } 28 \text{ ml}$

   $\text{SVR} = \dfrac{(87 - 10)80}{3.5} = 1760 \text{ dynes/sec/cm}^5$

   $\text{PVR} = \dfrac{(31 - 24)80}{3.5} = 160 \text{ dynes/sec/cm}^5$

   $\text{LVSW} = (100 - 24) \times 28 \times 0.0136 = 29 \text{ g-m/beat}$

   $\text{RVSW} = (40 - 10) \times 28 \times 0.0136 = 11 \text{ g-m/beat}$

   The CO and CI values are abnormally low and indicate the onset of clinical hypoperfusion. The high SVR indicates the body's attempt to maintain MAP. This high SVR means that Mr. C.'s injured heart is pumping against an abnormally high resistance, which increases myocardial oxygen demand. Since Mr. C.'s coronary circulation is obviously impaired, we must be concerned that he may not be able to meet these increased oxygen demands, and that this may result in further ischemia and infarction. LVSW is markedly decreased while RVSW remains within normal limits.

6. Appropriate aims at treatment would be:

   - To reduce SVR in an attempt to reduce myocardial oxygen demand and improve cardiac output

- To reduce Mr. C.'s PCWP to a value that promotes optimum left ventricular stroke work and cardiac output but avoids pulmonary congestion
- To improve myocardial contractility

These might be accomplished through the use of

- Afterload reduction with nitroprusside
- Diuretics (± nitroglycerin)
- Positive inotropic agent such as digoxin, dopamine or dobutamine. You must keep in mind that increasing contractility may increase myocardial oxygen demands which may lead to further myocardial damage.

IMPORTANT: The continued monitoring of hemodynamic parameters is necessary to assess the effectiveness of therapeutic intervention. The construction of ventricular function curves based on these data can further assist in guiding therapeutic interventions.

7. Nitroprusside has a very rapid onset of action and can cause a dramatic fall in blood pressure because of its potent vasodilating action.
8. The resulting reduction in SVR allowed the heart to pump more effectively so stroke volume and therefore cardiac output increased. This increase in cardiac output must have been sufficient to compensate for the fall in SVR, so MAP remained stable (MAP = CO × SVR).

Case 2

Mrs. B. is a 70-year-old woman who was admitted to the hospital 4 weeks ago with a fractured hip. Her past history indicates that she has been in good health previously, aside from mild hypertension.

Last night she developed severe chest pain and shortness of breath. She was transferred to the Intensive Care Unit. A 12-lead ECG was done and showed right bundle branch block and sinus tachycardia. As you come on shift, preparations are being made to insert a pulmonary artery catheter and arterial line.

1. What are the indications for hemodynamic monitoring in this case?

Upon insertion of the pulmonary artery catheter, the following pressures are obtained:

$$\overline{RA}: \qquad 18 \text{ mmHg}$$
$$PA \text{ systolic:} \qquad 55 \text{ mmHg}$$
$$PA \text{ diastolic:} \qquad 32 \text{ mmHg}$$
$$\overline{PA}: \qquad 40 \text{ mmHg}$$
$$PCWP: \qquad 8 \text{ mmHg}$$

Her vital signs at this time are BP 112/90 mmHg, HR 130 beats/min, respiration 30/min.

2. Interpret these results.

Thermodilution cardiac output determination is done and Mrs. B.'s CO is found to be 5.0 liters/min. Her BSA is 1.7 m².

3. Calculate her MAP, CI, SV, SVR, and PVR and interpret the results.

Diagnostic procedures are undertaken and the diagnosis of pulmonary embolism is confirmed.

4. What is the basis of treatment for pulmonary embolus?

Case 2 Answer Key

1. To distinguish between pulmonary embolism and acute myocardial infarction, both of which may present with the signs and symptoms demonstrated by Mrs. B.
2. The presence of high pulmonary artery pressure with a normal PCWP suggests a pulmonary problem as opposed to left-sided cardiac failure. The high $\overline{RA}$ pressure suggests right ventricular failure, which may be associated with pulmonary embolus. These hemodynamic parameters suggest that Mrs. B. may have experienced a pulmonary embolus.
3. $MAP = \dfrac{112 + 2(90) \text{ mmHg}}{3} = 97 \text{ mmHg}$

   $CI = 5.0 \text{ liters/min} \div 1.7 \text{ m}^2 = 2.9 \text{ liters/min/m}^2$

   $SV = 5.0 \text{ liters/min} \div 130 \text{ beats/min} = 0.038 \text{ liters, or 38 ml}$

   $SVR = \dfrac{(97 - 18)80}{5.0} = 1264 \text{ dynes/sec/cm}^5$

   $PVR = \dfrac{(40 - 8)80}{5.0} = 512 \text{ dynes/sec/cm}^5$

   The results support the possibility of pulmonary embolus. SVR is normal while PVR is markedly increased. CI and SV are on the low side of normal but she is maintaining an adequate MAP.
4. Supportive management of pain, hypoxia, and right heart failure. Removal of the embolus obstruction with agents such as streptokinase may be undertaken.

Case 3

Mr. I. is an 80-year-old man who was admitted to the Coronary Care Unit with an extensive anterior myocardial infarction. On admission he was short of breath and crackles were heard in both lung fields up to the midscapular regions. Chest x-ray confirmed the presence of pulmonary edema. He was given intravenous furosemide at that time. Several hours later he received another dose of IV furosemide for continued shortness of breath and bibasilar crackles. He improved following this and was placed on regular doses of furosemide and digoxin. A fluid restriction and low sodium diet were instituted.

Two days later you observe Mr. I. is becoming confused and disoriented. His blood pressure is 96/72 mmHg and his heart rate is 94 beats/min. His skin is cool and clammy. Checking his chart you note that his urine output has fallen to 10 ml/hr. His chest, however, is clear and he does not have distended jugular veins. A pulmonary artery catheter is inserted and thermodilution cardiac output determination is performed.

1. What is the purpose of inserting a pulmonary artery catheter in this patient?

His hemodynamic parameters are found to be:

BP:	92/70 mmHg
HR:	102 beats/min
RA:	1 mmHg
PA systolic:	20 mmHg
PA diastolic:	6 mmHg
$\overline{PA}$:	11 mmHg
PCWP:	3 mmHg
CO:	2.7 mmHg

(Mr. I. is 173 cm tall and weighs 72 kg.)

2. Calculate MAP, SV, CI, SVR, and PVR.
3. Interpret the measured and calculated hemodynamic parameters.
4. What are the aims of treatment in this case and how would they best be achieved?

Case 3 Answer Key

1. To determine whether Mr. I.'s hypoperfusion is due to cardiac failure or hypovolemia. It is often difficult to ascertain clinically whether the patient needs treatment to reduce preload and afterload or needs fluid replacement. Although the absence of such clinical signs as basilar crackles and elevated jugular venous pressure points to the need for fluid replacement, it is important to be certain. Giving fluid to a patient who is already in cardiac failure may further compromise his or her ventricular function. Another important reason for instituting hemodynamic monitoring in this case is to monitor therapeutic intervention.

2. $MAP = \dfrac{92 + 2(70)}{3} = 77$ mmHg

     $SV = 2.7$ liters/min $\div 102$ beats/min $= 0.026$ liters or, 26 ml

     $CI = 2.7$ liters/min $\div 1.85$ m^2 $= 1.46$ liters/min/m^2

     $SVR = \dfrac{(77 - 1)80}{2.7} = 2252$ dynes/sec/cm^5

     $PVR = \dfrac{(11 - 3)80}{2.7} = 237$ dynes/sec/cm^5

3. The low PCWP and $\overline{RA}$ indicate hypovolemia. The low SV goes along with hypovolemia, and the increased heart rate is an attempt to improve cardiac output. PVR is normal. SVR is elevated, as would be

expected, as a compensatory mechanism to maintain arterial blood pressure. Cardiac output and cardiac index indicate severe hypoperfusion. These hemodynamic parameters, along with the clinical findings, support the diagnosis of hypovolemia as the cause for Mr. I.'s hypoperfusion.

4. The aim of treatment is to improve cardiac output and perfusion by increasing preload. This can be achieved by careful volume replenishing with IV fluids. Continued hemodynamic monitoring is necessary to guide volume replacement and prevent fluid overload.

Case 4

Mr. W. is a 50-year-old male who was admitted to the Coronary Care Unit with an acute inferior myocardial infarction. Physical findings upon admission included cool, clammy skin, crackles to bases bilaterally, and a pansystolic murmur heard best at the apex and radiating to the left axilla. Upon insertion of a pulmonary artery catheter and arterial line the following parameters were obtained (BSA is 1.7 m²):

HR:	105 beats/min
RA:	12 mmHg
PA systolic:	50 mmHg
PA diastolic:	26 mmHg
PA:	34 mmHg
PCWP:	23 mmHg
BP:	105/85 mmHg
MAP:	92 mmHg
CO:	2.5 liters/min
SVR:	2560 dynes/sec/cm⁵

Large v waves were noted on the PCWP waveform tracing. These enlarged v waves, along with the physical findings, suggested a diagnosis of acute mitral regurgitation.

1. How would severe mitral regurgitation affect Mr. W.'s cardiac output?

In order to improve cardiac output, the treatment options would include:

a. Fluid administration
b. Inotropic agent administration
c. Afterload reduction (nitroprusside administration)

2. Comment on these treatment options as they would apply to Mr. W.'s case. Indicate whether each option is appropriate and give reasons for your answers.

Case 4 Answer Key

1. When the left ventricle contracts it will eject a portion of its output back up into the left atrium since the mitral valve is incompetent. Thus, the left ventricle must work harder to eject an adequate volume out into the aorta. In Mr. W.'s case, since his SVR is significantly elevated, the increased impedance to aortic flow further encourages back flow into the left atrium and cardiac output is further impaired.

2. a. This is not necessary because RA is adequate. (PCWP is high but is inaccurate due to the presence of large v waves.) More fluid at this point may strain the heart further and may make mitral regurgitation worse.

   b. This would increase myocardial contractility, but may also increase regurgitant flow. It may also, depending on the specific agent used, increase SVR and further increase the oxygen demands of Mr. W.'s recently infarcted myocardium.

   c. By decreasing the amount of resistance to aortic flow, it is possible to decrease the amount of regurgitant flow. Since a larger fraction of left ventricular output is ejected into the systemic circulation, cardiac output will increase. A decrease in afterload will also result in decreased myocardial oxygen demands. If cardiac output increases, heart rate may return to a normal level, further decreasing myocardial oxygen demand.

For these reasons afterload reduction would be the most appropriate therapeutic intervention. Careful monitoring of hemodynamic parameters with construction of ventricular function curves is necessary to guide treatment. The addition of inotropic agents may be indicated, in some cases in conjunction with afterload reduction to maximize cardiac output.

Case 5

Mrs. A. is a 68-year-old female who has been in hospital for the past 5 weeks recovering from a cerebrovascular accident. She has had a Foley catheter in place since admission. Last night she developed a temperature of 39.4°C, accompanied by chills, diaphoresis, and restlessness. Blood was drawn and sent for culture. Urine specimens were also sent for culture. She was given ASA suppositories. She did not improve over the next 2 hours and in the same period her blood pressure fell from 110/80 mmHg to 88/50 mmHg and her heart rate increased from 90 to 120 beats/min.

She was transferred to the Intensive Care Unit. Oxygen was given per mask and an intravenous line was established. A pulmonary artery catheter and an arterial line were inserted. The following hemodynamic parameters were obtained:

HR:	120 beats/min
BP:	88/50 mmHg
$\overline{\text{RA}}$:	1 mmHg
PA systolic:	16 mmHg
$\underline{\text{PA}}$ diastolic:	8 mmHg
$\overline{\text{PA}}$:	11 mmHg
PCWP:	3 mmHg
CO:	8.6 liters/min

1. Calculate MAP and SVR.
2. Interpret the results of the measured and calculated hemodynamic parameters.
3. What is the mechanism behind the abnormal CO and SVR values?
4. Mixed venous blood and arterial blood are drawn and analyzed for

oxygen content. The a-v DO_2 is significantly below normal. Give two reasons for this decreased a-v DO_2.
5. What are the aims of therapeutic intervention in this case and how might they be achieved?

Case 5 Answer Key

1. $$MAP = \frac{88 + 2(50)}{3} = 63 \text{ mmHg}$$

$$SVR = \frac{(63 - 1)80}{8.6} = 577 \text{ dynes/sec/cm}^5$$

2. The low PCWP and $\overline{RA}$ indicate low effective circulatory volume. The CO is markedly elevated and the SVR is markedly decreased. These parameters suggest that Mrs. A. is in septic shock.
3. The SVR is low due to the vasodilating effects of endotoxins and the release of kinins, serotonin and histamine that accompany septicemia. Since resistance to left ventricular ejection is so low, the heart is able to pump more blood, and cardiac output increases. The increased heart rate also helps elevate cardiac output.
4. The elevated cardiac output means that blood is passing through the systemic circulation more rapidly than normal, so less oxygen is being picked up by the tissues. In septic shock, shunting occurs at the microcapillary level. Because blood is being shunted away from capillary beds, the oxygen is not reaching the tissues and therefore is not being extracted normally.
5. At this stage the aim of therapy is to achieve and maintain a preload that will optimize cardiac output. This can be achieved through the administration of fluid to "fill up" the vascular compartment. It is also important to identify and treat the cause of the sepsis, thus eliminating the source of vasodilating stimuli.

Case 6

Mr. H. is a 49-year-old man who was admitted to the Coronary Care Unit with a diagnosis of acute anterior myocardial infarction. Upon admission his vital signs were

HR:	125 beats/min
BP:	90/62 mmHg
Respirations:	26/min

He denied chest pain at that time but complained of shortness of breath. His extremities were cool with faint radial and pedal pulses. Intravenous dopamine was initiated at 5 μg/kg/min and was increased to 7.5 μg/kg/min to bring his BP up to 110/74. His peripheral perfusion did not improve, however, and he became slightly confused. A pulmonary artery catheter and arterial line were inserted and a thermodilution cardiac output determination was performed. His hemodynamic parameters at this time were

HR:	128 beats/min
BP:	110/70 mmHg

RA:	9 mmHg
PA systolic:	43 mmHg
PA diastolic:	29 mmHg
$\overline{PA}$:	34 mmHg
PCWP:	26 mmHg
CO:	3.0 liters/min
SVR:	1973 dynes/sec/cm^5

1. What would you suggest be done to improve Mr. H.'s cardiac output and peripheral perfusion and why?

Nitroprusside is initiated at 0.5 μg/kg/min and slowly increased to 2 μg/kg/min over the next several hours. Mr. H.'s hemodynamic parameters (with dopamine at 7.5 μg/kg/min and nitroprusside at 2 μg/kg/min) are

HR:	90 beats/min
$\overline{BP}$:	104/70 mmHg
$\overline{RA}$:	8 mmHg
PA systolic:	41 mmHg
PA diastolic:	26 mmHg
$\overline{PA}$:	31 mmHg
PCWP:	23 mmHg
CO:	3.9 liters/min
SVR:	1497 dynes/sec/cm^5

Mr. H.'s peripheral perfusion improves somewhat and he is no longer confused. He remains slightly dyspneic and he continues to have crackles heard in both lungs. His urine output is 15 ml/hr. Since PCWP and $\overline{RA}$ pressures remain elevated, it is decided that his preload should be reduced to a more optimum level.

2. How would you reduce his preload?
3. How would you determine what Mr. H.'s optimum preload is?

Mr. H. is given intravenous furosemide and his hemodynamic parameters, including cardiac output, are repeated. His optimum PCWP is found to be 18 mmHg, at which time his cardiac output is 4.4 liters/min and his LVSW is 63 g-m/beat. (His HR is 88 beats/min and BP is 110/80 mmHg at this time.)

Case 6 Answer Key

1. Afterload reduction should be instituted. The use of dopamine alone may increase Mr. H.'s BP but it also increases his myocardial oxygen demands. Contractility is increased through the use of positive inotropic agents such as dopamine, but this means that the ventricle is beating more forcefully against a high resistance. Afterload reduction will reduce this resistance and allow an increase in stroke volume while decreasing myocardial oxygen demands.
2. Use of a diuretic agent such as furosemide would be appropriate in this case.

3. Construction of a ventricular function curve based on hemodynamic parameters obtained at different levels of PCWP. Hemodynamic monitoring should be continued during therapy with diuretics and the PCWP that corresponds with the best LVSW (or CO etc., depending on what parameter is used to evaluate left ventricular function) is the optimum level and should be maintained.

Section 3 Quiz

For each multiple choice question circle the letter that corresponds to the correct answer.

1. Therapeutic intervention for a patient with low stroke work and high wedge might be to:
    i. alter PCWP to achieve optimum stroke work
    ii. shift the ventricular function curve upwards
    iii. decrease afterload
    iv. decrease contractility
        a. i only
        b. ii only
        c. i, ii, and iii
        d. all of the above

2. One important use of ventricular function curves is to adjust the patient's PCWP to optimize:
    a. stroke work
    b. heart rate
    c. a-v DO_2
    d. CVP

3. A patient in a hyperdynamic state has a ventricular function curve that:
    i. is depressed
    ii. is augmented
    iii. shows high stroke volume
    iv. shows decreased stroke work
        a. ii only
        b. i and iv
        c. iii only
        d. ii and iii

4. In hypovolemic shock, you would usually see:
   i. decreased PCWP and $\overline{RA}$
   ii. decreased SVR
   iii. increased SVR
   iv. tachycardia
      a. iii only
      b. i, iii, and iv
      c. ii and iv
      d. i only

5. In the early stages of septic shock a hyperdynamic picture may be seen. Hemodynamic monitoring will show:
   a. decreased SVR and increased CO
   b. decreased SVR and decreased CO
   c. increased SVR and increased CO
   d. increased SVR and decreased CO

6. In the later stages of septic shock SVR may start to increase.
   a. true
   b. false

7. A patient with low effective circulatory volume, due either to blood loss or excessive vasodilation, will have a low PCWP.
   a. true
   b. false

8. a-v DO_2 is low in the later stages of septic shock.
   a. true
   b. false

9. Low cardiac output (as seen in cardiogenic shock) results in a decreased a-v DO_2 because blood remains in the capillaries for a relatively short time.
   a. true
   b. false

10. For a patient in severe cardiogenic shock, one aim of therapeutic intervention is to shift the ventricular function curve downwards.
   a. true
   b. false

11. Increasing the contractility of the failing left ventricle when it still has to pump against a very high afterload can further tax the already compromised myocardium.

 a. true
 b. false

12. Anaphylactic shock is caused by histamine release, which results in peripheral vasoconstriction.

 a. true
 b. false

13. Constructing a right ventricular function curve involves plotting:

 a. LVSW against PCWP
 b. RVSW against PCWP
 c. RVSW against $\overline{RA}$
 d. LVSW against $\overline{RA}$

14. Which of the following will usually shift the ventricular function curve upwards?

 a. Increasing PCWP to greater than 24 mmHg
 b. Decreasing contractility
 c. Decreasing preload
 d. Increasing contractility

15. In pulmonary embolism:

 a. PA systolic and diastolic are decreased, PCWP is increased
 b. PA systolic is increased, PA diastolic is decreased, PCWP is increased
 c. PA systolic and diastolic are normal, PCWP is increased
 d. PA systolic and diastole are increased, PCWP is usually normal

16. In severe cardiac tamponade:

 i. all intracardiac pressures may equalize
 ii. CO decreases
 iii. $\overline{RA}$ pressure increases during inspiration
 iv. MAP decreases during inspiration

 a. ii only
 b. i and ii
 c. all of the above
 d. none of the above

17. In ARDS:

   i. PCWP may be normal or low

   ii. protein leak results in decreased intravascular oncotic pressure

   iii. hydrostatic pressure within capillaries is usually high

   iv. PVR may be elevated

      a. i only

      b. i, ii, and iv

      c. ii, iii, and iv

      d. all of the above

18. Mechanical ventilation can result in:

      a. decreased venous return

      b. increased contractility

      c. negative intrathoracic pressure during inspiration

      d. none of the above

19. In mitral valve disease resulting in incomplete valve closures:

   i. blood is pushed back into the right atrium during systole

   ii. a large v wave may be seen in the PCWP tracing

   iii. PCWP is not representative of LVEDP

   iv. therapeutic intervention is aimed at reducing impedance to aortic blood flow

      a. i only

      b. i, ii, and iii

      c. ii, iii, and iv

      d. all of the above

20. In ventricular septal defect:

   i. blood is usually shunted from the left to right ventricles

   ii. left ventricular cardiac output may be reduced

   iii. RA pressure may increase

   iv. RA O_2 saturation is less than PA O_2 saturation

      a. i only

      b. i, ii, and iv

      c. iii only

      d. all of the above

21. In early septic shock, fluid administration is usually necessary to increase effective circulatory volume since extensive vasodilation occurs.

a. true
b. false

22. A patient has a CO of 9.0 liters/min and an SVR of 420 dynes/sec/cm^5. Cardiogenic shock may be suspected in this case.

a. true
b. false

23. Afterload reduction is often the treatment of choice in severe mitral regurgitation.

a. true
b. false

24. The use of dopamine can increase the contractility of infarcted myocardium.

a. true
b. false

25. Afterload reduction can increase cardiac output by reducing the resistance the left ventricle must pump against.

a. true
b. false

Section 3 Quiz Answers

The bracketed numbers following each answer indicate the pages where discussions for each question can be found.

1. c [80]	14. d [59]
2. a [58]	15. d [91]
3. d [81]	16. c [91]
4. b [83]	17. b [93]
5. a [84]	18. a [92]
6. a [85]	19. c [89]
7. a [83]	20. d [90]
8. a [85]	21. a [85]
9. b [86]	22. b [86]
10. b [86]	23. a [90]
11. a [86]	24. b [86]
12. b [84]	25. a [86]
13. c [59]	

If you had any incorrect answers, go back and review the areas with which you had difficulty. When you feel that you fully understand the material in Section 3, you are finished with this learning package. I hope it has helped you to review the pertinent aspects of hemodynamic monitoring, helped you to learn some new concepts, and, most of all, helped you to put together all this information so that it will be useful for you in the clinical setting. For those of you who want more information, many excellent resource books and articles are available. A list of pertinent reference readings is provided in the bibliography.

Section 3 References

1. Alonso DR, Scheidt S, Post N, et al: Pathophysiology of cardiogenic shock. Quantification of myocardial necrosis, clinical, pathologic, and electrocardiographic correlations. Circulation 48:588, 1973
2. American Edwards Laboratories: Understanding hemodynamic measurements made with the Swan Ganz catheter. Santa Ana, Calif: American Edwards Laboratories, 1979
3. Anderson CS: The pathophysiology of shock: An overview. In Guthrie M (ed): Shock. New York: Churchill Livingstone, 1982
4. Burg MB: Tubular chloride transport and the mode of action of some diuretics. Kidney Int 9:186, 1976
5. Chatterjee K, Parmley WW: The role of vasodilator therapy in heart failure. Prog Cardiovasc Dis 19:301, 1977
6. Chatterjee K, Parmley WW, Swan HJC, et al: Beneficial effects of vasodilator agents in severe mitral regurgitation due to dysfunction of subvalvular apparatus. Circulation 48:684, 1973
7. Dikshit K, Vyden JK, Forrester JS, et al: Renal and extrarenal hemodynamic effects of furosemide in congestive heart failure after acute myocardial infarction. N Engl J Med 288:1087, 1973
8. Edwards BR, Baer PG, Sutton RAL, et al: Micropuncture study of diuretic effects on sodium and calcium reabsorption in the dog nephron. J Clin Invest 52:2418, 1973
9. Ferrer MI, Bradley SE, Wheeler HO, et al: Some effects of nitroglycerine upon the splanchnic, pulmonary and systemic circulations. Circulation 33:357, 1966
10. Fewell JE, Abendschein DR, Carlson CJ, et al: Continuous positive-pressure ventilation does not alter ventricular pressure-volume relationships. Am J Physiol 240 (Heart Circ Physiol 9):H821, 1981
11. Fewell JE, Abendschein DR, Carlson CJ, et al: Mechanism of decreased right and left ventricular end-diastolic volumes during continuous positive-pressure ventilation in dogs. Circ Res 47:467, 1980
12. Fewell, JE, Abendschein DR, Carlson CJ, et al: Continuous positive pressure ventilation decreases right and left ventricular end-diastolic volumes in the dog. Circ Res 46:125, 1980
13. Forrestor JS, Diamond G, Chatterjee K, Swan HJC: Medical therapy of myocardial infarction by application of hemodynamic subjects. N Engl J Med 295:1404, 1976
14. Goldberg LI: Recent advances in pharmacology of catecholamines. Intensive Care Med 3:233, 1977

15. Goldberg LI: Cardiovascular and renal actions of dopamine: Potential clinical applications. Pharmacol Rev 24:1, 1972
16. Haynes JB, Carson SD, Whitney WP, et al: Positive end-expiratory pressure shifts left ventricular diastolic pressure-area curves. J Appl Physiol Respir Environ Exercise Physiol 48(4):670, 1980
17. Marini JJ, Culver BH, Butler J: Effect of positive end-expiratory pressure on canine ventricular function curves. J Appl Physiol Respir Environ Exercise Physiol 51(6):1367, 1981
18. Miller RR, Vismara LA, Williams DO, et al: Pharmacological mechanisms for left ventricular unloading in clinical congestive heart failure: Differential effects of nitroprusside, phentolamine, and nitroglycerine on cardiac function and peripheral circulation. Circ Res 39:127, 1976
19. Miller RR, Awan NA, Joye JA, et al: Combined dopanine and nitroprusside therapy in congestive heart failure. Circulation 55:881, 1977
20. Nagler AL, McCann R: The role of humoral factors in shock. In Ladingham IM (ed): Shock: Clinical and Experimental Aspects. New York: Exceprta Medica, 1976
21. Prewitt RM, Oppenheimer L, Sutherland JB, et al: Effect of positive end-expiratory pressure on left ventricular mechanics in patients with hypoxemic respiratory failure. Anaesthesiology 55(4):409, 1981
22. Rankin JS, Olsen GO, Arentzen CE, et al: The effects of airway pressure on cardiac function in intact dogs and man. Circulation 66(1):108, 1982
23. Rutherford RB, Buerk CA: The pathophysiology of trauma and shock. In Zuidema ED, Rutherford WF (eds): The Management of Trauma. Philadelphia: W. B. Saunders, 1979
24. Sibbald WJ: Bacteremia and endotoxemia: A discussion of their roles in the pathophysiology of gram-negative sepsis. Heart Lung 5:765, 1976
25. Smiseth OA, Refsum H, Tyberg JV: Pericardial pressure assessed by right atrial pressure: A basis for calculation of left ventricular transmural pressure. Am Heart J 108(3):603, 1984
26. Tyberg JV, Smith E, Smiseth O, et al: Assessment of left ventricular preload during PEEP from pulmonary capillary wedge pressure and right atrial pressure in dogs. Clin Invest Med 10 (Suppl 10):41, 1984
27. Sonnenblick EH, Frishman WH, LeJeontel TH: Dobutamine a new synthetic cardioactive sympathetic amine. Med Intelligence 300:17, 1979
28. Walinsky PL Acute hemodynamic monitoring. Heart Lung 6(5):838, 1977
29. Wiles JB, Cerra FB, Siegal JH, et al: The systemic septic response: Does the organism matter? Crit Care Med 8:55, 1980

Bibliography

JOURNAL ARTICLES

1. Abbot N, Walrath JM, Scanlon-Trump E: Infection related to physiological monitoring: venous and arterial catheter. Heart Lung 12(1):28, 1983
2. Baele PL, McMichan JC, March HM, et al: Continuous monitoring of mixed venous oxygen saturation in critically ill patients. Anesth Analges 61:513, 1982
3. Bodai BI, Holcroft JW: Use of pulmonary artery catheter in critically ill patient. Heart Lung 11(5):406, 1982
4. Dracup K, Brew C, Tillisch J: The physiologic basis of combined nitroprusside-dopamine therapy in post myocardial infarction heart failure. Heart Lung 10(1):114, 1981
5. Forrester JS, Diamond GA, Swan HJC: Corrective classification of clinical and hemodynamic function after acute myocardial infarction. Am J Cardiol 39:137, 1977
6. Gershen JA: Effect of positive end-expiratory pressure on pulmonary capillary wedge pressure. Heart Lung 12(1):28, 1983
7. Giboney GS: Ventricular septal defect. Heart Lung 12(3):292, 1983
8. Ganz W, Swan HJC: Measurement of blood flow by thermodilution. Am J Cardiol 29:241, 1972
9. Hudson-Civetta J, Carruthers Banner TE: Intravascular catheters: current guidelines for care and maintenance. Heart Lung 12(5):466, 1983
10. Jackson D, Everett J: A new method of fluid injection for cardiac output determination. Critical Care Nurse 67, Mar–Apr 1983
11. Kaye W: Invasive monitoring techniques. Heart Lung 12(4):408, 1983
12. Kaye W: Catheter and infusion-related sepsis: The nature of the problem and its prevention. Heart Lung 11(3):221, 1982
13. King E: Influence of mechanical ventilation and pulmonary disease on pulmonary artery pressure monitoring. CMA J 121:903, 1979
14. Nemens EJ, Woods SL: Normal fluctuations in pulmonary artery and pulmonary capillary wedge pressures in acutely ill patients. Heart Lung 11(5):393, 1982
15. Rossi P, et al: Short and long-term prognostic and functional stratification of acute myocardial infarction by hemodynamic and ergometric evaluation. Heart Lung 12(4):344, 1983
16. Runkel R, Burke L: Troubleshooting Swan Ganz catheters. Heart Lung 12(6):591, 1983

17. Sedlock S: Interprepation of hemodynamic pressures and recognition of complications. Critical Care Nurse 39, Nov–Dec, 1980
18. Shellock FC, Riedinger MS: Reproducibility and accuracy of using room-temperature vs ice-temperature injectate for thermodilution cardiac output determination. Heart Lung 12(2):175, 1983
19. Spence M, Lemberg L: Hemodynamic monitoring in the coronary care unit. Heart Lung 9(3):541, 1980

BOOKS

1. Berne RM, Levy MN: Cardiovascular Physiology, 4th ed. St. Louis, Mo: C. V. Mosby, 1981
2. Braunwald E, Ross J, Sonnenblick EH: Mechanisms of contraction of the Normal and Failing Heart, 2nd ed. Boston: Little, Brown, 1976
3. Ellerbe S (ed): Fluid and blood component therapy in the critically ill and injured. New York: Churchill Livingstone, 1981
4. Guthrie M (ed): Shock. New York: Churchill Livingstone, 1982
5. Guyton AC: Textbook of Medical Physiology, 6th ed. Philadelphia: W. B. Saunders, 1981
6. Karliner JS, Gregoratos G: Coronary Care. New York: Churchill Livingstone, 1981
7. Rushmer RF: Cardiovascular Dynamics. Philadelphia: W. B. Saunders, 1976

Glossary

afterload: Resistance to systolic ejection of blood out of the ventricle.

baroreceptors: Pressure receptors located at the carotid bifurcation and aortic arch that are involved in reflex mechanisms to maintain arterial blood pressure.

CAPP: Coronary artery perfusion pressure. Calculated as

$$CAPP = MAP - PCWP$$

cardiac index: Expression of cardiac output normalized by body surface area. Calculated as $CI = \dfrac{CO}{BSA}$

cardiac output: The amount of blood pumped by the heart per unit time (usually liters per minute).

chemoreceptors: Cells located in the aortic and carotid bodies that respond to changes in arterial oxygen and carbon dioxide content by influencing the vasomotor center.

chronotropic: Relating to the rate of myocardial contraction (heart rate).

compliance, ventricular: Diastolic tone or distensibility of the ventricular myocardium, the elasticity of the heart that allows it to stretch during ventricular filling.

contractility: Force of left ventricular contraction independent of the effects of preload and afterload. If force of contraction increases at constant preload and afterload, an increase in contractility is said to have occurred, e.g., effect of norepinephrine on myocardial cells.

CVP: Central venous pressure.

inotropic: Relating to the force of myocardial contraction.

LVEDP: Left ventricular end-diastolic pressure. Reflects left ventricular preload.

LVSW: Left ventricular stroke work. Calculated as

$$LVSW = (BP_{sys} - PCWP) \times SV \times 0.0136$$

MAP: Mean arterial pressure. Calculated as

$$MAP = \frac{SBP + 2DBP}{3}$$

where SBP is the systolic blood pressure and DBP is the diastolic blood pressure.

mean pressure: Time-averaged pressure. May be denoted by a line over the parameter, as in $\overline{RA}$ pressure.

MVO$_2$: Myocardial oxygen consumption.

overwedge: Overinflation of balloon on pulmonary artery catheter. Results in falsely elevated PA pressure readings.

oxygen consumption: Amount of oxygen consumed by the body per unit time (usually milliliters per minute).

oxygen saturation: Ratio of the actual oxygen content of hemoglobin and the total oxygen carrying capacity of the hemoglobin, expressed as a percentage.

$\overline{PA}$ pressure: Mean pulmonary artery pressure.

PCWP: Pulmonary capillary wedge pressure, which is an approximation of LVEDP. Also called pulmonary artery wedge pressure or pulmonary artery occlusion pressure.

preload: Myocardial fiber length at end diastole. Approximated by ventricular end-diastolic pressure. (True preload is actually best evaluated using transmural pressure.)

PVR: Pulmonary vascular resistance. Resistance to right ventricular ejection of blood into the pulmonary vasculature. Calculated as

$$PVR = \frac{(\overline{PA} - PCWP) \times 80}{CO}$$

$\overline{RA}$ pressure: Mean right atrial pressure.

RVEDP: Right ventricular end-diastolic pressure. Reflects right ventricular preload.

RVSW: Right ventricular stroke work. Calculated as

$$RVSW = (PA_{sys} - \overline{RA}) \times SV \times 0.0136$$

stroke volume: Amount of blood ejected by the ventricle per contraction. Calculated as

$$SV = \frac{CO}{HR}$$

stroke work: Measure of how hard the ventricle is working to eject blood.

SVR: Systemic vascular resistance. Resistance to left ventricular ejection of blood into the systemic circulation. Calculated as

$$SVR = \frac{(MAP - \overline{RA}) \times 80}{CO}$$

transmural pressure: End-diastolic pressure minus pericardial pressure. Best measure of preload.

Index

Italicized page numbers refer to figures.